Ketogenic Diet + Atkins Diet

Special 2 in 1 Bundle Edition!

Contents

Introduction

Much has been made of all sorts of quick-weight loss, and fad diets, all delivering the promise of a slimmer figure, glowing good looks, and good health forever and ever. Unfortunately, that is all that they deliver: PROMISES. The slimmer figure and good looks may last for a little while, but the good health facet may not even be achieved even if the weight loss objectives are met.

The problem with these diets is that they were only designed for short-term weight loss, and if we really want to talk about diets, we know that over 97% of dieters get back the pounds that they have lost, and in many cases, actually gain more than what they originally weighed in the first place!

That is for only one diet - people spend a lot of their time going on diets, and the results are hardly successful. In a 2007 study, it was learned that women spend, on the average, 31 years of their lives going on a diet; just exceeding the number of years that men spend, 28.

Another problem with diets is that they usually require a drastic change in the eating patterns. Many require a dramatic drop in caloric intake. Some diets require that people eat tasteless and unappealing foods, making them want to end their diets quickly, and they just revert to their old eating patterns.

The diet that I will lead you through, Ketogenic Diet, is not a fad diet, and its underlying principles have been around for decades. In fact, Ketogenic Diet has not only been a sure-fire approach to weight loss. It has been used to treat certain health conditions, and help others avoid various illnesses.

Our Ketogenic Diet journey will be an educational one on nutrition and diet, and ultimately, a ticket to a better body, and glowing health. This book is divided into two parts, with Part I (Chapters 1 to 4) providing a background on the nutrition and health aspects of any diet. In Chapter 1, we will look at the roles of fat, carbohydrates, and protein in our nutrition, including a history of how humans have regressed to increasing rates of obesity, heart disease, and metabolic problems.

In Chapter 2, we look at how the human body uses the foods that we eat, and convert them into energy and tissue. Chapter 3 describes the body's descent into obesity, including the role of carbohydrates in this sometimes deadly process. We will talk about the various ailments and diseases that arise from a nutrition program with faulty information and premises. In Chapter 4, we review the concept of ketogenesis in detail, including the mechanics of how and why ketones are produced.

Part II of the book (Chapters 5 to 8,) will discuss the how to's for starting on, and progressing with Ketogenic Diet. Chapter 5 will discuss the objectives of the diet, including the significance of ketosis, and provide dieting patterns and schedule to follow. Chapter 6 will detail what foods should be eaten in the diet, and what should be avoided.

Chapter 7 will discuss the basic pointers on how to succeed on the diet. On the flipside, the chapter will also point out what traps to avoid. Chapter 8 gets down to the real world of Ketogenic Diet: Actual recipes that will provide you with a week's worth of meals, snacks, and even desserts, with an emphasis on getting you on a tasty and flavorful track to a healthier life style.

Ketogenic Diet has had a growing number of devotees and fans because of the documented success of millions who have tried it. There are also a growing number of health professionals, including M.D.'s and dieticians who have gone public in promoting the benefits of Ketogenic Diet.

A growing number of nutritionists have also began to assail the prescribed "balanced" diets that continue to be endorsed by official, national and international medical associations and even, governments. Many Ketogenic Diet devotees now dismiss these official pronouncements as downright wrong, and even, dangerous.

In this book, we will set the record straight on dietary fat and more precisely, its role in the human health and well-being. We will see that dietary fat deserves to be elevated as THE food nutrient of choice, and should be consumed in at least equal quantities, as carbohydrates and proteins. Fat is not only recommended, but required, as a component of healthy eating and well-being, to help assure you a life of optimal vitality and health!

PART I – BACKGROUND INFORMATION
Chapter 1. The False Promises of Carbohydrates

Mankind's original fuel

All engines need fuel and energy, and human beings, as the most complicated naturally-occurring engine in existence, is no exception. While we put gasoline as fuel in cars, as human beings, we also need to have our own fuel, and this fuel is food. More precisely, food that will be needed in relatively large amounts, consumed consistently and regularly.

Our fuel, food, is comprised of three basic macronutrients: carbohydrates, fat and protein. Everything we eat as fuel for storage and energy comes from these three macronutrients. The human body needs these to function properly. How has the consumption of macronutrients changed over the last 10,000 years or so and what has brought us to this world of dieting and more correctly, failures in dieting?

Gog

Let me introduce you to "Gog," a typical ancestor from our prehistoric days, from about 10,000 years ago, give or take a few hundred years. Gog was a male member of the most advanced and latest version of homo sapien, of which we eventually became the proud descendants. In that stage of human history, Gog was part of that group called the "hunter-gatherers," who sourced their food from animals that they hunted and killed, and from fruits or berries that they happened to come across in their hunting adventures.

Gog and other co-inhabitants of the planet at that time subsisted on a diet that consisted mostly of animal fats, protein, and fibrous berries and fruits. Their

Vitamin D source was principally the sun, and they had little use for plant carbohydrates, from whose chlorophyll content merely transfers the sun's Vitamin D nutrients.

Gog stayed out in the sun for most of the day, and the sun provided his "D". Vitamin D was, and continues to be important to sustain the human's bodily functions, but it is clear that fat was to be the human's primary source of fuel.

It is important to note that even today; certain tribes and cultures subsist on essentially high-fat diets and thrive with robust health. The Maasai group in Africa and Eskimos are modern day cultures that are known for the very small part that carbohydrates play in their diet. These groups are sustained by high fat diets in particularly unforgiving weather conditions. Apparently, their low-carbohydrate lifestyles have turned their metabolisms around to fat burners, rather than glucose burners.

This low-carbohydrate situation seemed to be the way that nature designed humans and their fuel needs: Man got their energy from fat, and fat was their fuel. For millions of years, the genius of nature, or even the genius of a Creator deemed that fat would be man's primary source of energy.

Was this simple diet enough for Gog's sustenance and health? For this, we can look at the archaeological record. On the next page, we present a table that shows life expectancy from the year 9,000 B.C., when agriculture, tilling the soil for carbohydrate foods, is generally is known to have started.

TABLE 1.

Life Expectancy of Our "Lithic Ancestors"

Period of Time	Ave. height-male	Ave. height-female	Life expectancy-Male	Life expectancy-Female
30,000 to 9,000 B.C. (Meat and fat is about 2/3 of the diet)	177.1 (5'9.7)	166.5 (5'5.6)	35.4	30.0
9,000 to 7,000 B.C. (Some agriculture already started – Meat and fat is now less than 1/3 of the diet)	172.5 (5'7.9)	159.7 (5'2.9)	33.5	31.3
7,000 to 5,000 B.C. (Agriculture	169.6 (5'6.8)	155.5 (5'1.2)	33.6	29.8

spreads widely in the Early Neolithic age – Meat is now 30% of the diet)				
5,000 to 3,000 B.C. ("Late Neolithic," i.e., the transition towards full blown agriculture is mostly complete)	161.3 (5'3.5)	154.3 (5'0.7)	33.1	29.2
3,000 to 2,000 B.C. (Early Bronze Era)	166.3 (5'5.4)	152.9 (5'0.2)	33.6	29.4

The above table shows that when humanity began the agricultural stage, life expectancy actually decreased! The decrease should actually have been bigger if we factor in the increased physical security that our ancestors had because of agriculture: enclosed communities and better defensive mechanisms and positions against predatory animals. In fact, deaths from predators on the general population would be reduced to almost zero, with fatalities coming from predators only occurring with the armed male hordes that elected to hunt for animals.

Gog consumed just what his body required, and most of what he consumed was fat from whatever animals he hunted down. The fat he consumed was burned immediately and quickly, not because of physical activity per se, but because the human body, unlike a car, consumes and uses up energy even while he is in a state of rest and even sleep.

From Chapter 2, we will learn that the carbohydrates he consumed were immediately expended for quick bursts of energy. Gog therefore used his nutrients efficiently and effectively, not requiring much fat to be manufactured or stored. This is something we will come back to later in Chapter 4, when we talk about the mechanics of the diet.

"Post" Gog

The archaeological record also shows that as agriculture began to produce more food, agricultural plant products began to play a bigger role in the human diet. When human beings retreated into safer and cozier settlements, there was less of a need to go out and secure animal foods for food. Also note from the table, that males had higher life expectancies than females, even when their lives appeared to be in more mortal danger, being the hunters.

Humans, especially the male hunters, often turned into prey for the animals of the day. Despite this, males still had higher life expectancies because they presumably ate more of the fat that they hunted, possible consuming much of their meat immediately after securing them, and even before distributing them to their waiting families.

In a couple of thousand years more, meat, and especially fat, would continue to take a backseat to processed carbohydrates. Agriculture would become more efficient, and humans would not only produce more of carbohydrate foods, especially in the form of wheat and rice, they could store these foods longer!

For example, wheat and rice could be pounded down to flour, and stored in silos and bins over long periods of time. Because they could be stored longer, they became a much cheaper and more available source of sustenance and nutrition. After all, why risk lives hunting for food when it could be retrieved in a matter of minutes from a storage bin?

Health problems increase

As time marched on, life expectancies would increase as humankind learned more about medicines, while infant mortality rates would plummet. By the Middle Ages, average life expectancies would approach 50 years or so, but other mortal problems would surface: obesity, heart disease, and metabolic issues. Increased carbohydrate intake would totally throw human metabolic processes into crisis.

Before we get into the science and chemistry of food, we can historically trace these problems to one thing: Humans stopped eating naturally, and more importantly, reduced their intake of fat. Millions of years of eating unprocessed foods and fat were in the millennial blink of an eye, overturned, and the human body was shocked, and not pleasantly, to the new nutritional realities. Natural and fat was out, processed and carbohydrates were in. So-called blood diseases, and all sorts of unidentified diseases, presumably cancer and diabetes, began to spread.

Modern Man Doubles Down on the Carbohydrate Problem

From the middle ages to well into the 20th century, humankind saw an increasing, if not alarming incidence of heart disease and symptoms reflecting diabetes. Archaeologists, who have studied heart disease not surprisingly, found that heart disease was extremely rare in pre-industrial societies. After the so-called

"Industrial Revolution," which gave witness to large-scale mechanization, heart and metabolic diseases shot up, and people were all of a sudden getting sick in newer ways. Heart attacks and symptoms attributable to strokes suddenly took hold.

Modern conventional wisdom, however, attributed this rise in diseases to the sedentary lifestyle that the advances in technology, especially the invention of machines, brought. The thinking was people were getting fatter and sicker, not because of food, but because people were doing less manual labor than from thousands of years ago. "Experts" assumed that fat deposits formed because people didn't exercise or were sitting, or lying around more.

What they missed or ignored was how human diet was drastically transformed when agriculture took over the human food supply. Modern technology not only made people move around less, it also helped mass produce agricultural products at a faster and cheaper pace.

After wheat and rice were produced in huge, mass proportions, sugar production finally became widespread in the 1700's, and made food, especially, carbohydrates, taste much better. Well into the 1900's, foods high in processed carbohydrate content, such as pizza, French fries, candies, and processed dairy foods gained shot up in popularity.

Moreover, processed carbohydrates became popular because of the short amount of time required to prepare, and with the advent of the microwave oven, cook them. Fast food became a symbol of modern society, and these foods are mostly all about carbohydrates in most of its forms: popcorn, potato chips, and candy bars being the most widespread and popular.

The growth of carbohydrates was largely ignored as a cause of increased heart disease. Because the true villain for human health was being overlooked, a boogeyman had to be found or invented – dietary fat.

Fat gets a bad rap

Sometime in the 1990s, fat was beginning to get demonized. It quickly became the dirty word of the nutrition industry and it was fashionable to shun as a deadly health hazard. Doctors derided it as a scourge to physical well-being, and consumers followed the medical herd, making fat as the primary source of a bunch of physical ailments, most of them revolving around the heart. High "bad" cholesterol, weight gain, artery disease, you name it – all of these were blamed on fat.

The curious thing about the demonization of fat was that there wasn't (and there still isn't) adequate scientific proof to back up these claims of nutritional Armageddon arising from fat.

Despite what science failed to prove, everyone jumped on the low-fat bandwagon, consuming mass quantities of food that, while indeed lacking fat, were instead, loaded with carbohydrates, especially sugar. The results of this "diet revolution" were that the average American got more obese, and the rate of increase of heart problems hastened.

According to U.S. Department of Health and Human Services statistics, by 2001, roughly a third of the American population was already overweight. This, of course, came with the increase in the incidence of heart disease and diabetes also soared.

The result of this "conventional wisdom" was that fresh whole foods such as meat, eggs, and their fatty components—the foods our ancestors ate for centuries—were being quickly replaced with low-fat "Frankenfoods" such as margarine, low-fat snack cookies, and skim milk. These foods were not only full of sugar and carbohydrates; some were also loaded with artificial ingredients. When these substances are consumed regularly, over time, the human body reacts by gaining weight, showing symptoms of fatigue and brain fog, and succumbing to chronic conditions.

Although scientific research produced findings to the contrary, fat—especially saturated fat—had developed a lasting reputation for being bad. Although the low-fat diet craze eventually dwindled, the damage was done. Fat was shunned and carbohydrates were placed on the nutritional pedestal.

In fact, government authorities began to promote, and still promote, the consumption of mostly carbohydrates, for their recommended dietary combinations. The National Institutes of Health, for example, continue to suggest that 70% of a diet should be comprised of carbohydrates in various forms. Subsequently, in the "Dietary Guidelines for America, 2015-2020," issued by the U.S. Department of Agriculture, dietary fats are merely mentioned almost as a footnote as oils.

The USDA also says that food oils (not fat) are limited to fat in liquid form, while naming vegetable cooking oils as the only source of fat nutrients that should be available for human consumption. There is no mention of the animal fat that our ancestors like Gog consumed, which was actually the main source of his energy fuel. The USDA caps their dismissal of fat by allowing very limited consumption levels of animal fat for the "ideal" diet.

To disseminate this fat-starved diet, the USDA pictorialized their concept of an ideal diet with the "My Plate" diagram, which portrays this dismissal of animal fat from the daily diet. The "Plate" emphasizes vegetables, fruits, grains, and protein, and assigns dairy as a supplemental item on the plate diagram. This diagram suggests that at least sixty percent of a person's recommended calorie intake should be comprised of foods from carbohydrates, which make up grains, vegetables, and fruits.

Fats from non-aquatic animals as beef, pork, and lamb, have been excluded in the nutritional conversation, with the "Plate" admonishing everyone to shun the so-called "trans-fat". Government agencies' objective is to limit the consumption of red meat, cheese, and processed meats.

The USDA recommended "Plate" is depicted as follows:

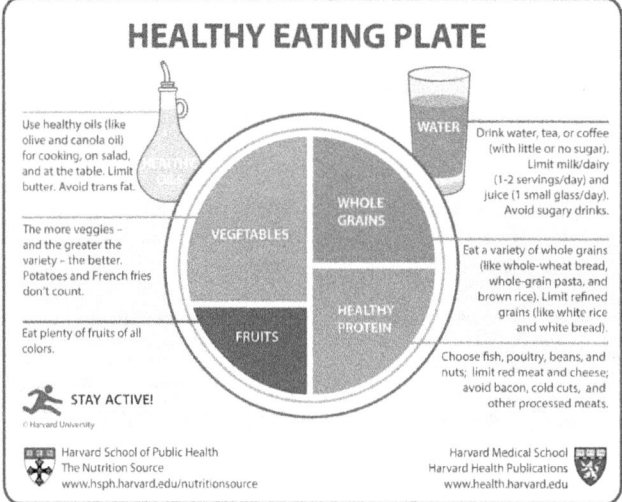

Source: U.S. Department of Agriculture

Nevertheless, many current scientific studies have not only repudiated the omission of animal fats from the diet, but have argued that fat from animals is not just a necessary component of the human diet, but should be accepted as the largest part of human nutrition. This is especially true when someone is endeavoring to lose weight, and eventually, get healthier.

The USDA, the National Institutes of Health, the World Health Organization, our grandparents, physicians, and even our gym instructors have been telling us what to eat. Now after we have followed their recommendations, and of course, our own palate, we consume the food and enjoy them. Sometimes, we don't really enjoy these, but just follow the herd to appear to stay modern and in touch. Regardless of what we eat, certain things happen in our body to convert all those goodies into energy.

Chapter 2. The Chemistry of Eating

In Chapter 1, we mentioned that food is the fuel that provides human beings with energy. The three macronutrients, carbohydrates, protein, and of course, fat are the fuels that power our bodies 24/7, day in and day out, whether we are moving around, resting, or even sleeping. In this chapter, we see the role of the macronutrients in the sustenance of our bodies, and how food is converted into fuel and other substances in our body.

Our bodies are highly intelligent, and yet, "needy" machines. They know exactly what they want, and more importantly, what they need. The most unconscious of these needs, and yet probably the most important, is the need for fuel to provide our bodies with energy. Without these energy sources, our cells would starve to death.

You see all these shows and movies about people stranded in islands, forests, and deserts without food? Those are the consequences when your conscious minds and bodies cannot get the fuel necessary to function, and endure.

The first step, the easy and conscious part; chewing and swallowing, puts food into our bodies. The next, more important, however subconscious step; happens inside our body -- to break down this food for absorption, and conversion into energy. This process is called metabolism.

Eating up

Metabolism describes the chemical reactions that take place to maintain the dynamic state of our bodies and their constituent cells. Metabolism has two subordinate bodily functions to process the food/fuel, which we can conveniently divide into the following:

Catabolism – This refers to the breakdown of the molecules that we ingest. The macronutrients are broken down in substances and molecules that can be usable for the body to convert into fuel and energy.

Anabolism - This refers to the amalgamation of all compounds needed by the human body. Basically, in this stage, the body takes what has been broken down by catabolism, and processes the molecules to convert them to energy.

When we ingest the foods that contain the macronutrients of carbohydrates, fat, and proteins, our bodies immediately begin to work on the foods that we take in. The last conscious effort we have in this process is the swallowing of the foods that we have either chewed or drunk. When the mass of chewed food and/or liquids have passed our throat, and heads down our esophagus, the rest of body takes over beyond our conscious control. What happens to these foods?

In order to make sure that it always has access to energy; our body has several metabolic pathways it can use to convert the food that we eat into useable energy, and energy that we can store. We will summarize what these metabolic pathways are all about in the rest of this chapter.

For human beings, the default metabolic pathway is one that uses the glucose from carbohydrates as fuel. As long as you provide your body with carbohydrates, it will use them as energy, and storing excess macronutrients as fat in the process. When you deny your body of carbohydrates, it has to turn somewhere else to get the energy it needs to live. For millions of years up to about 9,000 years ago, the human body turned to mostly, stored and dietary fat.

Anabolism– fed and fasting states

In the metabolic process, a distinction also has to be made between the "fed" and the "fasting" state when the nutrients are being broken down during the anabolic stage. The fed state occurs about 4 hours after eating a meal or snack. This is the time when the body begins to absorb the digested nutrients. Some of these nutrients, especially carbohydrate-based ones, are used to meet immediate energy needs, while converting the extra nutrients to energy stored products.

In the "fasting state," which occurs 4 or more hours after eating, the body uses fat as its main source of energy. How fat or thin we are, depends on how much of fat stores are used, and of course, how those stores are built.

Let us now discuss these blessed little fuel sources.

Carbohydrates

These are probably the tastiest of all foods, the "lightest" on the mouth and the palate, the easiest to swallow, and from an economic standpoint, the cheapest. Rice and wheat for example, can be expanded to 2 or 3 times their original uncooked mass, then laced and mixed with all manner of sugars, creams, flavors, and texturized ingredients to provide the tastiest satisfaction from the lips to the tongue.

After we ingest carbohydrates, these are immediately broken down, by the introduction of various enzymes, into glucose, which is basically blood sugar. Some of the glucose is burned for instant energy, but usually, there is excess glucose left in the blood stream to trigger the body to try to regulate these increases in glucose.

Glucose is the body's favorite source of energy on demand, and is the fuel of choice for athletes, bodybuilders, and gym rats. This is why we have "sugar boosts" after consuming an energy bar or cookie, after a workout or an athletic exercise. The metabolic process that glucose undergoes is called "glycolysis," where the glucose is converted to mostly glycogen.

In the human body's infinite wisdom, it knows that too much glucose can be a problem (which we will see in a while.) To regulate the level of blood sugar, the body lets the pancreas release insulin, a regulating hormone. From this we can see that nature has considered carbohydrates to be inherently bad for the human body, otherwise, why limit it?

Indeed, nature has planted an organ in our body, the pancreas, to produce a singular hormone, insulin, to prevent the body from taking on too much blood sugar. We will visit insulin again in the next chapter when we talk about the effects of sugar and fat on the body.

Proteins

Proteins are responsible for creating the "building blocks" of our body tissues. The most common forms are lean meats and certain legumes. The foods containing protein provide more of a "chewing" sensation before being swallowed, provide the most "filling" sensation, and are more expensive per ounce, than carbohydrates.

Proteins are broken down into amino acids, and used by body cells to form either new proteins or to mixed up in some kind of amino acid "pool". This pool serves like a cache for the molecules, creating some sort of reservoir. Amino acids comprise a significant percentage of our body mass. A big percentage of our cells, tissues, and muscles are also comprised of amino acids.

Amino acids, therefore, perform a bunch of key body functions. One of the most paramount is giving our cells their form and structure. The metabolic process that protein undergoes is called "transamination," where the amino acids we eat are converted to glycogen or other protein compounds.

Aside from forming body tissues, amino acids play an important part in the storage and transport of essential nutrients. They have significant influence over the functions of arteries, glands, organs, and connective tissues, such as tendons. They also are indispensable for repairing tissues, and healing wounds, most especially in the skin, hair, bones, and muscles. Proteins also play an important role in the elimination of various waste deposits arising from metabolism.

Just as ingesting too much of carbohydrates is an issue, the body will need to "dispose" of "extra" amino acids produced over and above the body's requirements. The excess amino acids are transformed by enzymes in the liver into urea and keto acids. These keto acids can then be utilized as extra sources of energy, and via different anabolic processes, are transformed into glucose, or stored in the muscles as fat. Urine and sweat takes care of eliminating urea from the body.

Fat

Fat can be yummy, and can be gross at the same time, but fat is the king of human body fuels; nature having decreed it as the best source of energy. Fat from foods usually is ingested as part of other food items. For example, one can eat the fatty part of steaks, the skin of chickens, and the fat from fish, and egg yolks. Pure fat can be taken in limited forms: of such foods as whole milk and fried eggs.

When fats are eaten, they are converted into fatty acids and glycerol. They are digested in the person's small intestine. They are then turned into lipoproteins for different essential functions (we will talk about bad and good cholesterol, LDL and HDL in the next chapter).

Getting energy from carbohydrates, proteins, and fat

When you eat, the nutrient molecules are absorbed in the intestine and into the bloodstream. In the fasting state, the cells will soon be taking up these nutrients and chemically burn them to liberate energy. The most common chemical fuel is the sugar glucose. Other molecules, such as fats or proteins, can also supply energy, but they usually have to first be converted to glucose or some intermediate that can be used in glucose metabolism.

This is where the energy superstar, adenosine triphosphate, or ATP, comes in. After all the three macronutrients are metabolized, ATP, a critical element in human metabolism, is produced when the body burns the sugars together with other nutrients. Mitochondria in the cells convert the food that we eat into ATP, which is a comparatively smaller molecule which functions as "energy intermediate" when we metabolize food.

ATP is often referred to as "chemical currency" as the body uses it as a direct energy source. The body produces ATP when it burns up various nutrients and sugars, while our cells ingest ATP when engaging in actions such as producing movement, and on an atomic scale, building larger molecules. Our cells then chemically process ATP, resulting in the release of energy, in order for the human body to engage in various activities.

In essence, our body cells take out the chemical energy from different nutrient molecules such as proteins and carbohydrates, and then utilize this chemical energy to produce ATP. How do we go from glucose to ATP? This is achieved through the process of "oxidation".

For example, glucose, the molecule that came from our consumption of carbohydrates, including many dietary sugars and starch, are broken down to make waste products like water and carbon dioxide. But our cells will utilize the energy freed up from breaking down a single glucose molecule, and produce about thirty ATP molecules.

As soon as a cell has produced ATP, it will now utilize the ATP to meet any of its energy requirements. Cells require energy in order to produce large molecules, such as hormones, for example. Muscle cells also make ATP to generate movement. As a cell produces a large molecule, ATP molecules are broken down. The cell utilizes this energy to produce original bonds among smaller molecules resulting in the production of a bigger one, and the process goes on.

All these processes occur amazingly without our conscious effort or thinking. Our bodies are amazing machines that do all these processes automatically. If we take in the right foods in the right amounts, there shouldn't be any problems.

However, since the age of agriculture dawned on humanity 9,000 years ago or so, our bodies have unfortunately, not been so lucky.

Chapter 3. How We Get Fat and Sickness From Food

We now have an idea of how the body processes the macronutrients. Let us pay attention to the negative side of eating, and what happens when we take in too much of the "wrong" types of food into our bodies, especially carbohydrates. In the previous chapter, we mentioned that our bodies were "intelligent" in the singular sense that it tells us when we need fuel, and signals our bodies to take in food whenever our energy sources are getting low.

On the flipside, however, our bodies cannot be "smart enough" to totally withstand bad nutrition, which is eating foods that were not originally designed for our consumption. Despite our bodies' best "efforts," we become obese and sick, and there is very little that it can do from a self-defense standpoint to fight this. In nutrition, the worst thing that can happen to the human body, aside from not being fed enough, is being fed too much, and worse, being fed too much of the wrong foods.

The sugar curse

It may seem that carbohydrates, especially sugars, will be demonized in this, and other books, as the benefits of low-carb, high-fat diets continue to portray as the correct way towards proper weight loss and good health. Actually, as we have seen in the previous chapter, sugar by itself, is not the problem. In fact, we talked about the importance of glucose, and how even proteins and fats are broken down to make sugar in the body.

Glucose is absolutely essential to life, and our metabolism cannot function properly without it. Each cell in our body is able to utilize glucose as energy.

Even when we cannot obtain glucose from our diet directly, we can get what we need from fats and proteins. In fact, we have a constant supply of it in our bloodstream. But it can also create severe problems.

Too much sugar

We have discussed how processed carbohydrates, because of their lower price, accessibility, and taste, have become the most consumed macronutrient. The fact that they are also the "lightest" on the mouth and the palate, added to carbohydrates' promotion as the preferred macronutrient, it has practically ensured that human beings will eat them more than any other food.

But sugary and carbohydrate-packed foods are also the most easily converted and metabolized macronutrient. They pass through the digestive tract the fastest, and these factors combined ensure that too much of carbohydrates can be eaten, especially if the habit is picked up when we are young. The bottom line is that anytime we fill our bodies with more than the needed fuel levels, the storage capacity of our liver for sugar is exceeded, and sometimes, greatly.

The liver can store up to only around 5% of its mass as glycogen, which has been converted from excess glucose. When the liver is packed at close to full capacity, the excess sugars are transformed by the liver into more fatty acids.

Worse, these fatty acids go back into the bloodstream, and is distributed throughout our bodies and stored as fat! These fats are stored away where our bodies are designed to store these as adipose fat cells. These areas include, but not limited to, the popular regions of the butt, breasts and hips for women, and the stomach for men. These fatty cells can also imbed themselves in the arteries, causing arteries to deteriorate and being clogged with fat and debris from extra fat.

As a disastrous reverse bonus, as soon as these areas become full with fatty tissues and adipose cells, they will start to leak over into our vital organs – these include the kidneys, liver, and heart. The presence of fat will impair and impede the organ's ability to perform, raise blood pressure, lower metabolic rates, cause a feeling of constant tiredness, and expose the body to illness and sickness as our immune system is weakened.

The body pushes excess glucose into the cells to be made into ATP, or stored as glycogen which are converted into fat droplets called triglycerides in the fat cells, or adipose tissue. "New fat" has just been created.

The wrong sugars

Compounding the "too much" sugar problem is that we may not only be eating too much of carbohydrates, but humans, more than ever, are consuming the wrong carbohydrates. "Gog" and our prehistoric ancestors filled their bellies with natural berries, natural wild fruit, and natural fibers. The operative was natural, and Gog only ate foods that nature provided.

Today, however, there are a vast multitude of foods that contain sugars that nature did not intend us to ingest. Many foods, especially desserts, have sugar (sucrose) and high fructose corn syrup. These are sweetening agents that help enhance the taste of many foods and drinks – practically all non-diet sodas and ice creams contain them.

These are very different from natural sugars that contain glucose, which is an essential life giving nutrient, taken in the right quantities, but fructose is another matter. The molecule is not part of our normal metabolism and we do not produce it. A tiny fraction of cells in the human body can make use of it except liver cells. Since these cannot be properly assimilated into other cellular functions, they get turned to fat, and are eventually secreted into the blood.

Insulin and the Big D- Diabetes

We mentioned in the previous chapter that our bodies are intelligent enough to know that carbohydrates, and especially, processed sugars, are not good for the body, and it takes great pains to try to mitigate the effects of bad dietary habits. One of its best defense mechanisms is the pancreas, which secretes insulin to help mitigate the creation of too much blood sugars and fats, the results of which can be devastating, as we have seen above.

Insulin plays an indispensable role in the body. Its biggest role is its interaction with glucose to let our bodies utilize glucose properly as energy. The pancreas, the organ which produces insulin, excretes enough insulin and it acts as some sort of a "key" that allows the cells of the body to take in, and use glucose as energy.

Insulin assists in controlling blood glucose levels by alerting muscle cells, fat cells, and the liver to extract glucose from the blood. If our bodies have sufficient energy, insulin alerts our liver to process the incoming glucose, and store it as glycogen.

The glucose that insulin "pushes" in to the cells in the form of glycogen can then be transformed into ATP, or stored as fat as described earlier. This additional stored glycogen can then be utilized later on when the body needs more energy. When our bodies experience a disruption in the balance between fat production and the secretion of insulin, diabetes will occur.

Type1 Diabetes

This form of diabetes has also been called insulin-dependent diabetes or juvenile-onset diabetes, and accounts for less than 10 percent of all diabetes cases. Usually a genetic affliction, in this diabetes type, our body's immune system kills the cells that are responsible for releasing insulin, which in effect, stops insulin production.

Type 2 Diabetes

This is the type that Ketogenic Diet will most likely try to address. Type 2 diabetes is the most common form of diabetes (over 90% of diabetes cases), and is usually the result of a diet with very high in carbohydrates. The ones suffering the disease will manifest any symptom prior to diagnosis. Usually Type 2 diabetes is found during adulthood, although a few cases have been known to have been diagnosed in children.

In this affliction, our bodies cannot process insulin the right way. While the most common root cause is still debatable, there is a growing consensus that this is a "lifestyle" disease emanating from an overconsumption of carbohydrates. The bottom line is that the ability of the body to produce insulin has been overwhelmed by the amount of glucose produced. This condition is called, "insulin resistance," and eventually, the body will make less and less insulin, leading some to require insulin injections.

Since Type 2 Diabetes is a lifestyle disease, the way to deal with it is to change our lifestyles! This is best done by going on Ketogenic Diet, and getting the body into the ketosis state.

Chapter 4. Ketosis and Ketogenesis

The human body was designed to use fat for energy, and when mostly fat is used for energy, it does not store that fat, and the body becomes lean, as nature designed it. From Chapter 2, we found out that our bodies have several metabolic pathways it can use to convert the food that we eat into useable energy. The default metabolic pathway is one that uses the glucose from carbohydrates as fuel. As long as you provide your body with carbohydrates, it will use them as energy, storing fat in the process.

When you deny your body with carbohydrates, it has to turn somewhere else to get the energy it needs to live. If you starve your body of carbohydrates, therefore, the body will burn fat, and in the metabolic process, it will produce something called, "ketones." These are what may save your life!

Ketones are organic compounds that are made in the liver from fatty acids, and are generated from the breakdown of fats, especially when the body cannot "locate" any glucose to turn into energy. Ketones are formed almost as a defensive action by the body. When it "senses" that there is not enough sugar or glucose to provide for the body's energy needs, it immediately creates an alternative fuel source.

The Creation of Ketones and Ketosis

During times of fasting, or when we intentionally follow a low-carbohydrate diet, it turns to fat for energy. In simple terms, fat is taken to the liver where it is broken down into glycerol and fatty acids through a process called beta-oxidation. The fatty acid molecules are further broken down through a process called ketogenesis, and a specific ketone body called acetoacetate is formed.

If we continue on Ketogenic Diet, over time, our bodies will adapt to using ketones as fuel, and our muscles will convert the acetoacetate into beta-hydroxybutyrate or BHB. BHB is actually the preferred ketogenic source of energy for your brain, and acetone, most of which is expelled from the body as waste.

When dietary carbohydrates are suddenly taken away from the diet, more fatty acids are released from fat cells, which leads to more fat cells being burned up in our liver. This increase in the burning of fatty acids in the liver eventually causes ketone bodies to be produced, and induces ketosis, a new metabolic state.

Other hormones are likewise affected, and these help transfer the use of this new fuel, instead of carbohydrates, to body tissues. The majority of calories burned up by the human body will now come from this fat breakdown.

The glycerol created during the beta-oxidation process enters into a stage called gluconeogenesis. During gluconeogenesis, the body converts glycerol into glucose that your body can use for energy. Your body can also convert excess protein into glucose. Your body does need some glucose to function, but it doesn't need carbohydrates to get it. In other words, during this period, our body is beginning to now burn fat instead of converted sugar! Ketosis has set in, and hopefully for good!

So is fat and ketosis bad?
Ketogenic Diet has been at the forefront of a big diet "revolution" for the past few decades. Its popularity continues to increase, as new scientific evidence continues to surface, and proves that fat does not deserve the bad nutritional reputation it has received. Is fat bad?

The human body was designed to use fat for energy, no matter where it is produced. This results in a lean body, as nature originally designed it. How does a dieter on Ketogenic Diet get to ketosis? Getting to a state of ketosis means ingesting less than 50 grams of carbohydrates per day, and in the next Chapters we will find out how to count these carbohydrates, including the tools you need to measure carbohydrate intake.

Weight loss in Ketogenic Diet

Now that you understand how your body creates energy and how ketones are formed, you may be still wondering just how this translates into weight loss. Let's provide a quick review and summary.

When you eat a lot of carbohydrates, your body happily burns them for energy and stores any excess as glycogen in your liver, or as triglycerides in your fat cells. When we take carbohydrates out of the equation or reduce our intake of them drastically, our body depletes its glycogen stores in the liver and muscles and then turns to fat for energy.

When our bodies start to burn stored fat, our fat cells shrink and you begin to lose weight and become leaner. Smaller, leaner cells = smaller, leaner bodies!

Ketosis has sometimes been confused with ketoacidosis, which is a pre-existing condition present in some diabetic patients. It is a condition where there is not enough insulin produced in the body. Ketosis is not ketoacidosis, and vice-versa. Ketosis will not lead to ketoacidosis, and assuming you have no other medical conditions that may prevent you from going on Ketogenic Diet.

While many people try to dismiss Ketogenic Diet as a dangerous fad diet, it is well worth noting that the diet has many helpful, life-changing, and life-saving effects on our bodies and long-term health. Weight loss and looking great is sometimes viewed as merely side benefits by those who have stayed on the diet for an extended period of time.

There are other ways on how Ketogenic Diet can contribute to your well-being and long life. If you understand what amazing benefits are in store, it will be very easy to get convinced to stay on the diet. Described below are the foremost benefits of going on Ketogenic Diet.

Elimination of Type-II diabetes

We mentioned that Type-II diabetes is a lifestyle issue, and that it can be cured by a lifestyle change. For diabetes, the best lifestyle change is to get on Ketogenic Diet, and stop letting carbohydrates ruin your health. Many Type-II diabetes conditions are treatable before requiring the use of injected insulin.

Reduction of the symptoms of epilepsy

Ketogenic Diet is sometimes recommended to help control seizure symptoms in some patients afflicted with epilepsy. Ketogenic Diet is prescribed by a doctor and the patient undergoes careful monitoring under the watch of a professional dietitian.

Reduction in the symptoms of cancer

Cancer cells are very much not like our healthy cells. One way that they have known to be way different is that they have about ten times as many more insulin receptors on their surface as ordinary cells. The receptors allow the cells to feed on nutrients and glucose coming from the bloodstream at a very significant rate.

The more carbohydrates that are catabolized, the more glucose are produced which helps the cancer cells gorge for their "nutrition." If we are able to remove carbohydrates from our diets, we can possibly deny cancer cells from their energy source.

Reducing the incidence and severity of Parkinson's disease and Alzheimer's

Parkinson's disease is one of those "motor system" disorders where the onset happens between the ages of 50 and 65 years old. In the United States, about 1 percent of people in that age group are affected with it. In Parkinson's disease, the dopamine-producing cells in the brain are seemingly destroyed. The symptoms of Parkinson's disease include slowness of movement, trouble with balance, tremors, and shaking.

Near the terminal phase, the victim is usually on a wheelchair, or bed-ridden. These symptoms show up after up to 80 percent of the dopamine-producing cells in the brain are devastated. While it is not exactly clear on how Ketogenic Diet can alleviate the symptoms of Parkinson's disease, it is highly possible that ketones, which have an anti-inflammatory effect on the brain, may be able to fix impaired neurons.

The ketones may also possibly bypass the area in the brain that is damaged, and bring much-needed energy to other areas in the brain.

Reduction of symptoms of Mitochondrial Disorders

Mitochondria are organelles that are of significant numbers in most human cells. This is where the essential biochemical processes of energy production and respiration take place. Mitochondria are also considered as the energy centers of the human body. They convert the food that we eat to adenosine triphosphate, or ATP, as we have learned in Chapter 2.

When mitochondria become dysfunctional, the cells are denied of the energy they need. Because the brain, muscles, heart, nervous system, and eyes demand the most energy, their cells are often the most significantly affected with a mitochondrial disorder. Affecting these body parts cause learning and intellectual disabilities, muscle weakness, hearing and visual impairment, respiratory disorders, and even seizures. There is no cure for mitochondrial disorders, so their treatment focuses on alleviating its symptoms and improving the quality of life of the sufferer.

Proper diet is often the first stage of therapy for these disorders, and with seizures are a common symptom, a high-fat, Ketogenic Diet is often part of the treatment plan.

Reduction of symptoms of Lou Gehrig's or ALS Disease

ALS (Amyotrophic Lateral Sclerosis) is a progressive, neuro-degenerative ailment that assaults the nerve cells in the spinal cord and brain. ALS specifically affects the motor neurons, which are responsible for voluntary muscle movement. When motor neurons die, they are no longer able to send nerve signals to the muscle fibers leading to slurred speech, difficulty swallowing, muscle weakness, and almost instantly fatal breathing. At any rate, most of the muscles begin to waste away, and the person affected becomes weaker.

The exact cause of ALS is unknown, and there is no cure for the disease. Researchers believe that disruptions of the mitochondria in the brain and changes in a person's diet may help those with ALS, as well. Studies on mice and other animals show that those under Ketogenic Diet experienced a greater decrease in symptoms than those who weren't.

Improved Focus and Mental Clarity

For the brain, exposure to too much glucose can result in neurotoxicity or the exposure of the nervous system to toxic substances. Many mental issues, such as brain fog and problems with memory, are caused by this condition. In Ketogenic Diet, the reduction of the supply of glucose diminishes the levels of toxicity in the body as brain starts to use ketones as fuel. Possible results are the ability to think more clearly, better focus, and better memory recall.

Increased Energy

When the body breaks down fat instead of carbohydrates, more energy is produced for each ounce of fat used, leaving the Ketogenic dieter with a feeling of heightened alertness and increased energy.

Better heart and coronary health

When there are less fat cells flowing through the blood stream, that means that there is less strain on the heart and the arteries. This is a result of less plaque clogging up the bloodstream, and a better functioning circulatory system.

Lower "bad cholesterol" levels

Weight and fat loss are the objectives of an overwhelming majority of people going on Ketogenic Diet. Of course, the associated benefits of a slimmer body can also lead to a decrease in "bad" cholesterol levels, blood pressure, and just better heart health.

Breaking the myths surrounding high fat diets

It is useful to know what people, even health professionals, can say to scare people from Ketogenic Diet. There are many myths and misconceptions that have surrounded, and clouded ketosis and Ketogenic Diet.

Ketosis myths

Myth 1: Carbohydrates are an essential nutrient for good health.

Myth2: Eating a low-carbohydrate diet can lead to vitamin deficiencies, especially Vitamin C, which come from carbohydrate-rich sugary fruits and vegetables.

Myth 3: Ketogenic Diet causes your body to go into ketoacidosis, which is dangerous.

Myth 4: Your kidneys will sustain damage from high fat consumption.

Myth 5: A high-fat diet will lead to osteoporosis, because it will cause the body to excrete calcium.

Myth 6: Eating fat makes you fat.

Myth 7: Ketogenic Diet leaves out carbohydrates completely.

Myth 8: Cholesterol from animal fat causes heart diseases.

PART II – Ketogenic Diet
Chapter 5. Ketogenic Diet Basics

Before we get into the nitty-gritty of the diet, an important few words on how Ketogenic Diet is different from other low-carbohydrate diets on the market.

Atkins Diet

Atkins Diet was at the forefront of the low carbohydrate revolution and brought ketosis and ketogenesis into public awareness about fifty years ago. Atkins Diet allows for a moderate amount of protein in the menu. The allowable ratio is about 50-35-15 in terms of fat/protein/carbohydrate ratio. In Ketogenic Diet, the overwhelming amount of calories should come from fat, about 70%.

Atkins Diet also puts a lot of emphasis on the two week, "induction" phase, where the dieter will have to consume the required macronutrients. Atkins Diet promoters claim that a person can lose up to fifteen pounds on the first week of the diet.

Atkins Diet also allows the dieter to slowly reintroduce certain carbohydrates after the induction period. On Ketogenic Diet, the dieters need to be on a high fat diet for the rest of their lives.

Paleolithic Diet

Paleolithic Diet focuses on the foods supposedly eaten by our prehistoric ancestors, just like Ketogenic Diet, and also reduces the emphasis on carbohydrates. But Paleolithic Diet also allows for more significant portions of vegetables and certain fruits. Certain grains are allowed, and in fact recommended. Like Ketogenic Diet, Paleolithic Diet forbids tubers and sweet potatoes. The big difference between both diets is that high fat dairy products can be consumed on Ketogenic Diet, but is expressly disallowed on Paleolithic Diet.

Other diets that promote lower carbohydrate intake

Two other famous diets, Zone Diet and South Beach Diet, also recommend carbohydrate intake significantly lower than that of Ketogenic Diet. However, they allow for the consumption of a wider variety of carbohydrates. Ultimately, only Ketogenic Diet dictates that the significant majority of macronutrients consumed should be from fat.

The importance of macronutrients

Our body's overwhelming source of fuel is the food that we eat. Some of our energy comes from sunlight (Vitamin D), but 99% of our fuel comes from macronutrients in the food that we eat. Ketogenic Diet's effectiveness depends almost wholly on what we eat and drink. There is no need for supplementation, such as vitamins when we go on Ketogenic Diet.

Think of the macronutrients as the gasoline that we put in our cars. Taking in the wrong macronutrients can be compared with putting contaminated fuel in your gas tank, or putting diesel fuel, for example, in a car that requires high-octane gasoline.

In Ketogenic Diet, the proper fuel is fat.

Getting on Ketogenic Diet

a. Prepare your household and cupboard for Ketogenic Diet

Going on a high-fat diet means a big change in lifestyle. If we are not living alone, and have to share our cupboards, refrigerators, and shopping budgets with other people, we need to properly announce that things will be changing drastically in the food storage department.

On Ketogenic Diet, carbohydrates are the big enemy, and we have to make sure that no "stealth carbs" manage to intrude our food space. Be organized, create lists, and shop carefully. We go into much greater detail on what we need to eat in the next chapter.

<u>b. How many grams of protein, carbs and fats should be eaten in Ketogenic Diet?</u>

In Chapter 1, we mentioned that most "authorities" recommend that about two thirds of calories should come from carbohydrates. This means that for a typical daily diet of 2,000 calories consumed, at least 1,300 calories of the total should be consumed in the form of carbohydrates. Additionally, around 500 calories should come from protein, and the remainder, should come from incidental, and trace quantities of fat.

Remember that these so called authorities do not even contemplate fat as being a food group, but only gives some token credit to fats as oils added to foods for taste and use in food preparation.

Ketogenic Diet turns this all around. Dietary fat should now make up about two-thirds of daily calorie consumption, allowing a maximum of ten percent to come from carbohydrates. Converting this to food weights, this means that under Ketogenic Diet, we should only consume daily between 30 and 50 grams of carbohydrates.

The more active a person is, however, a little more carbohydrates are added, maybe up to 100 grams, can be eaten. This is a concession to the fact that carbohydrates are useful for those that require short-term bursts of energy, such as those who go to a gym or exercise regularly and athletes.

For protein, the recommended quantity can be between 115 grams and 175 grams per day. The rest of the diet should be concentrated on fat. For a 2,000 calorie daily diet, we need to ingest at least 60%, or 1,200 calories of fat, 25%, or 500 calories from protein, and 15%, or 300 calories, from carbohydrates.

A note on protein which we have given very little attention to: Proteins are important in the creation, maintenance, and repair of muscle tissues. We want protein to rebuild our tissue, and not be an inefficient source of energy. In fact, excess proteins can turn into fat, the way carbohydrates are converted.

c. Recording and monitoring calorie and macronutrient intake

To ensure of the success of the diet, we need to carefully monitor how much of each macronutrient we are consuming daily, to ensure that the right proportion of calories are being consumed.

There are a multitude of carbohydrate/calorie counters that are available. The preeminent source is the suite of Atkins Diet publications that pioneered the high-fat revolution. These need to be purchased in publication or app form.

A good source to look for apps is http://www.mydreamshape.com/carb-counter-apps/

Regardless of whether you record your progress in a written journal, or monitor yourself via computer, tablet, or phone, you need to strictly be in compliance with the percentages I have just mentioned. This monitoring is especially important in the first few weeks, when you are transitioning your body into the ketosis state.

Of course, you need to pay strict attention to the actual macronutrients you can (and should not!) consume when you are on the diet.

d. Signs That You Are in Ketosis

Signs that you're in ketosis may start appearing after only one week of following a true Ketogenic Diet. For some people, it can take longer—as much as three months. The amount of time it takes for you to start seeing signs that your body is burning fat for fuel largely depend on you as an individual. When signs do start to show, they are pretty similar across the board.

<u>"Keto Flu"</u>

"Keto flu" or "low-carb flu" commonly affects people in the first few days of starting Ketogenic Diet. Of course, Ketogenic Diet doesn't actually cause the flu, but the phenomenon is given the term because its symptoms closely resemble that of the flu. It would be more accurate to refer to this stage as a carbohydrate withdrawal, because that's really what it is.

When you take carbohydrates away, it causes altered hormonal states and electrolyte imbalances that are responsible for the associated symptoms. The basic symptoms include headache, nausea, upset stomach, sleepiness, fatigue, abdominal cramps, diarrhea, and lack of mental clarity, or what is commonly referred to as "brain fog."

Carbohydrate addiction is a real thing. Some research shows that carbohydrates activate certain stimuli in the brain that can be dependence-forming and cause addiction. Carbohydrate addicts have uncontrollable cravings for carbohydrates, and when they do eat them, they tend to binge. For a carbohydrate addict, the removal of carbohydrates can cause withdrawal symptoms, such as dizziness, irritability, and intense cravings.

The duration of the symptoms varies—it depends on you as an individual, but typically "keto flu" lasts anywhere from a couple of days to a week. In rare cases, it can last up to two weeks. Some of the symptoms of the "keto flu" are associated with dehydration, because in the beginning stages of ketosis you lose a lot of water weight.

With that lost fluid, you also lose electrolytes. You can replenish these electrolytes by drinking enhanced waters (but make sure they are not sweetened) and drinking lots of homemade bone broth. This may help lessen the severity of the symptoms.

<u>Bad Breath</u>

Unfortunately, bad breath is another early sign that you're in ketosis. When you're in ketosis, your body creates acetone as a waste product. Some of this acetone is released in your breath, giving it a fruity or ammonia-like quality. You can combat bad breath by chewing on fresh mint leaves and drinking plenty of water, since bad breath is also associated with dehydration.

Decreased Appetite and Nausea

As your body adapts to Ketogenic Diet, you may have a decreased appetite. This is because you're providing your body with plenty of fat and protein, which are both highly satiating, and not a lot of carbohydrates. The nausea associated with "keto flu" can also decrease your appetite. When you reach this stage, it's important that you eat even if you feel like you aren't hungry. You want to make sure your body is getting enough calories and nutrients, especially in this time of transition.

Increased Energy

When the fog begins to clear and your body starts to become keto-adapted, the uncomfortable symptoms you were feeling will dissipate and you'll begin to see the benefits of following Ketogenic Diet. One of the first beneficial signs many people experience is an increase in energy. When your body breaks down fat instead of carbohydrates, more energy is produced gram for gram, leaving you feeling alert and energized.

Other Possible Signs

Cold hands and feet

Increased urinary frequency

Difficulty sleeping

Metallic taste in the mouth

Dry mouth

Increased thirst

Chapter 6. What to Eat. And What Not to!

Shopping for the right foods is the first and most important step short of putting the right food in the mouth. For today's food shopper, fortunately, most food manufacturers are sensitive to the needs and requirements of people who go on special diets such as Ketogenic Diet. In labeling their foods, they have endeavored to be more accurate and responsive to people who need the proper information to go on their diets.

Regardless of whether foods are "allowed," the serious dieter will still have to make sure that they are staying well within the required macronutrient ratios (preferably 65% fat, 20% protein, and 15% carbohydrates). If measuring ratios are not possible during a given meal, the overriding principle is that the majority of the calories eaten daily should come from fat, and a very small percentage should be from carbohydrates.

Quality

The "quality" of your food matters, especially when it comes to fat and protein sources. Going back to the prehistoric time, our ancestors got healthy on unprocessed and unrefined food alone. It would be healthy and beneficial if a diet plan replicates that prehistoric food profile. A Ketogenic dieter should also try to purchase foods that have the following descriptions on the labels: organic, grass-fed, free-range, and/or pasture-raised.

Food with labels that say, "farm-raised" should be avoided as much as possible, because in all probability, whatever has been "raised" in those "farms" have been sprinkled with a healthy dose of chemicals and preservatives to improve yield and increase the animals' sizes.

Meats, poultry, and seafood

These are the staples of Ketogenic Diet, not vegetables, rice, or grains. They are the most plentiful, and in fact, appetizing components of the diet, and contains naturally-occurring fat. There are many foods in this group that most people can eat all they want every day. Foods included in this food group comprise all types of beef, chicken, turkey, duck, fish, lamb, pork, shrimp, crab, and lobster.

Of course, "exotic" varieties such as ostrich, goat, deer, and buffalo, are also allowed, if available. While bacon and sausage are excellent sources of protein and fat, care should be taken in eating processed meats, especially hotdogs and sausages. Many brands contain substantial quantities of carbohydrate fillers.

Remember that when eating meat, make sure to stay within your recommended protein grams for the day, since your body converts excess protein into glucose via glucogenesis, which can kick you out of the ketosis state.

In the following lists, we will show what the carbohydrate and fat contents are for a particular food item. Remember that these measurements are for uncooked and undressed food. Because Ketogenic Diet is ultimately a low-carbohydrate diet, we are listing the carbohydrate content of each food item. We will also list the number of calories for each item. Note that there may be many varieties of food types, especially in the meat items, because meat comes from various parts of the animal.

The list below is a fairly large general representation of foods that we generally eat. In the reference section of this book, I provide some resources for carbohydrate and calorie counting, in general.

a. Foods that are good for Ketogenic Diet

Animal Meats:

Beef/Veal – 3 oz. has 0 carbohydrates, and about 300 calories

Pork - 3 oz. has 0 carbohydrates, and about 200 calories

Lamb - 3 oz. has 0 carbohydrates, and about 175 calories

Goat - 3 oz. has 0 carbohydrates, and about 100 calories

Venison -3 oz. has 0 carbohydrates, and about 150 calories

Other wild game:

Keep in mind, the organic and grass-fed meat. Even if they are a little more expensive, they are the healthiest options, because there is a much lesser chance that they will contain growth hormones and preservatives. Game meat has generally less calories than regular pork and beef, and for the most part, has zero carbohydrates.

Processed meats:

While being basically comprised of the same meats that we have just listed that have zero carbohydrates, the curing and processing required to give them taste, sometimes necessitates the adding of carbohydrates.

Bacon – 3 oz. has less than 2 grams of carbohydrates, and about 450 calories

Bologna – 12-gram slice has about 1 gram of carbohydrates, and about 50 calories

Pork rinds - 3 oz. has 0 carbohydrates, and about 300 calories

Salami - 12-gram slice has about 1 gram of carbohydrates, and about 50 calories

Sausage (e.g., Bratwurst, Kielbasa, etc.) - 3 oz. has 2 grams of carbohydrates, and about 300 calories

Make sure that these yummy meats do not contain added sugars or excess preservatives.

Poultry:

You can be liberal with the skin and the fat portions. There is no need to skim them off anymore. Once again, organic and grass-fed cuts are the healthiest options. These include:

Chicken – 100 grams has 0 carbohydrates, and about 120 calories

Duck - 100 grams has 0 carbohydrates, and about 130 calories

Goose - 100 grams has 0 carbohydrates, and about 160 calories

Ostrich - 100 grams has 0 carbohydrates, and about 110 calories

Pigeon -100 grams has 0 carbohydrates, and about 200 calories

Quail - 100 grams has 0 carbohydrates, and about 150 calories

Turkey - 100 grams has 0 carbohydrates, and about 125 calories

Speaking of poultry, eggs, especially the yolk part, are highly recommended. Organic eggs or eggs from grass-fed chickens are preferred.

Fish – fatty varieties, especially:

Bass - 100 g has 0 carbohydrates, and about 150 calories

Halibut - 100 g has 0 carbohydrates, and about 110 calories

Mackerel - 100 g has 0 carbohydrates, and about 200 calories

Salmon - 100 g has 0 carbohydrates, and about 140 calories

Tuna - 100 g has 0 carbohydrates, and about 150 calories

Trout - 100 g has 0 carbohydrates, and about 150 calories

Peanut Butter – Check the labels to ensure that the variety is very low in carbohydrates, and have no sugar content. 2 tbsps. of such varieties have about 5 g of carbohydrates, and 200 calories.

Dairy:

Butter – o carbohydrates and 500 calories per 100 grams

Cheese – Make sure that you watch out for blends! They may have sugars and other dangerous chemicals and preservatives to make them look, and taste like real cheese. Most well-prepared cheese without any fillers 100 g has 1.5 g carbs, and about 400 calories

Plant products:

Asparagus, green – 1 cup has 5 g of carbohydrates and calories

Avocados - 1 cup has 20 g of carbohydrates and 300 calories

Bamboo shoots - 1 cup has 8 g of carbohydrates and 40 calories

Broccoli - 1 cup has 6 g of carbohydrates and 30 calories

Celery stalks - 1 cup has 4 g of carbohydrates and 15 calories

Coconuts – 1 cup has 12 g of carbohydrates and 300 calories

Green, leafy vegetables, such as bok choy, lettuce, Swiss card, radicchio, endives. These are non-starchy vegetables and typically 1 cup has about 5-10 g of carbohydrates and between 25-50 calories.

Kale - 1 cup has 5 g of carbohydrates and 30 calories

Kohlrabi - 1 cup has 8 g of carbohydrates and 40 calories

Radish - 1 cup has 2 g of carbohydrates and 15 calories

Broth, especially self-made bone broth, non-sweet pickles, kimchee, sauerkraut, and mustard.

Almost all herbs and spices (no sweeteners and preservatives) and recipe enhancers such as lime juice, lemon, and their grated skins.

Whey protein - keep away from those with sugar, chemical additives, and soy additives

Nuts (make sure there are no sugar-based additives) such as Brazil nuts, hazelnuts, pecans, walnuts, sunflower seeds, sesame and pumpkin seeds, pistachios, pine nuts, and peanuts.

Oils such as coconut oil, pure lard, and olive oil

b. Take the following in moderation

These can be eaten after the initial phase of ketosis has been completed.

Plants:

Bell peppers, shallots, tomatoes - 1 cup has between 10-20 g of carbohydrates and 30-50 calories

Berry varieties, including strawberries, blackberries, cranberries, raspberries, and blueberries. Berries are tricky because while they have an abundance of sugars, they are rich in fiber, which greatly reduces their "net" carbs, or carbohydrates discounted by the fiber they contain.

Cabbage, cauliflower, broccoli, fennel, rutabaga, turnips, Brussels sprouts, and eggplant

Eggplant - 1 cup has 5 g of carbohydrates and 20 calories

Garlic -1 teaspoon has 1 g of carbohydrates and 4 calories

Leeks – The bulbs and lower leaf portions - 1 cup has 15 g of carbohydrates and 50 calories

Mushrooms - 1 cup has 2 g of carbohydrates and 15 calories

Olives - 1 cup has 5 g of carbohydrates and 20 calories

Rhubarb - 1 cup has 5 g of carbohydrates and 20 calories

Onion - 1 cup has 10 g of carbohydrates and 40 calories

Other Peppers- 1 cup has 10 g of carbohydrates and 40 calories

c. Foods that should be avoided at all costs

Alcohol in most forms. Most pure rums and some vodkas though, have zero carbohydrates. Bar beverages and alcohol-based drinks usually have a lot of sugars and syrups and should be avoided.

However, dieters can also consume a variety of beverages in moderation, as long as they contain no sugar. Check the labels carefully on so-called diet sodas to make sure that they do not contain any sugar. Unlimited drinks will include tea, coffee, and heavy cream, minus any refined sugars or sweeteners.

As with most diet plans, water is still the best bet as a beverage alternative. It is a good idea to drink at least half of your body weight in ounces. Plain water can be infused with fresh herbs, such as mint or basil, to provide a little variety. Sodas, flavored waters, sweetened teas, sweetened lemonade, and fruit juices should be avoided.

High-fructose corn-syrup is that deadly stealth sweetener found in most soft drinks, and juices. We mentioned fructose briefly in Chapter 2. If the "high" in high-fructose is not enough to scare someone away, consider that it also functions like a preservative, meaning that not only does it lack B vitamins and other important nutrients, it is chock-full of chemicals that have no business being in the human body.

Avoid grains and sugars in all of their forms. Grains include wheat, barley, rice, rye, sorghum, and anything made from these products. This means that Ketogenic Diet will have no breads, pasta, crackers, and rice. Sugar and anything that contains sugar is also not allowed. This includes white sugar, brown sugar, honey, maple syrup, corn syrup, and brown rice syrup.

There are many names for sugar on the ingredient lists. It's extremely beneficial to familiarize yourself with these names so you will know when a product contains sugar in any form. Be careful of artificial sweeteners like Splenda that could actually be made out of sucralose, which contains carbohydrates.

Breads, including wheat bread

Breakfast cereals

Chocolate bars and candies

Desserts, especially cakes, pies, and pastries

Energy bars, including protein bars

Energy boost drinks - look for sugarless varieties though

Ice cream

Oils that are processed are generally harmful to the body, and will impede Ketogenic progress. These include margarine, sunflower, cottonseed, safflower, canola, grape seed, soybean, and corn oils.

Pancakes and waffles

Rice

Sodas and sugary drinks, including most juice drinks

Syrups and chocolate toppings

T.V. dinners

The basic rule is this: You have to avoid foods and drinks with sugars, carbohydrates, and chemicals.

Chapter 7. Do's and Don'ts

While Ketogenic Diet can provide some awesome benefits, there are many pitfalls to avoid if one is to have success, and even avoid serious hazards to your health.

Mistakes on going on Ketogenic Diet

Because Ketogenic Diet is a radical departure from what most people are used to, it is easy to make mistakes. The following are the most common mistakes that can remove the benefits of Ketogenic Diet, and may even cause harm to your body:

1. To gain the maximum benefits from the diet, you have to be in a state of ketosis for at least two weeks. You CANNOT deviate from this, or you will basically need to start from zero again.

2. Eating too much processed fats and proteins. This is especially true for boxed or T.V. dinners. While they may have a lot of fat content, there are usually a lot of hidden sugars, and worse, artificial chemicals that can derail your progress.

3. Eating more protein as opposed to fat. Fat is the main source of energy, and eating excess protein is bad, because some of it is converted to sugar.

4. Being afraid of fat. In the dietary world, fat is a friend, and we need to forget all the misconceptions about it.

5. Not getting enough water. Sometimes we drink water to accompany carbs, especially sweets, so drastically reducing carbs may cause us to consume less water. Water is the most important element of any diet, and it sometimes helps to give the body a feeling of "fullness."

Chapter 8. Happy Keto Eating Recipes

Meal Plan for Ketogenic Diet

Congratulations! You've gone this far, and now it's time to be rewarded for your persistence and attentiveness.

This chapter will present 7 days' worth of Ketogenic-friendly meals and snacks, which will contain the bare minimum of carbohydrates, while maximizing the consumption of fats and fatty foods. Eating a combination of the meals will guarantee that you will consume less than 50 grams of carbohydrates per day, and should provide a pretty clear picture of the direction that needs to be taken in order to be successful on the diet.   Ketogenic Diet requires this proportion in order for the body to achieve ketosis quickly and consistently.

Breakfast Recipes:

1. Ketogenic Breakfast Muffins

Fat Ingredients:

1 medium Egg

1/4 cup Heavy Cream

1 slice cooked Bacon (Cured, Pan-Fried, Cooked)

1 oz. Cheddar Cheese

Other Ingredients:

Salt & Black Pepper (to taste)

How to Prepare:

1. Preheat oven to 350 F.

2. In a bowl, whisk the eggs with the cream and salt and pepper.

3. Spread into pam sprayed muffin tins, and fill the cups 1/2 full.

4. Place 1 slice of crumbled bacon to each muffin and then 1/2 oz. cheese on top of each muffin.

5. Bake for about 15-20 minutes or until slightly browned.

6. Add another 1/2 oz. of cheese onto each muffin and broil until cheese is slightly browned. Enjoy!

2. Ultra Ketogenic Style Egg Breakfast (Serves 2)

Fat Ingredients:

6 organic eggs

½ cup of heavy cream

1 tablespoon of butter

Other Ingredients:

1 cup of shredded spinach

A small pinch Sea Salt+ ground white pepper

1 small onion finely minced

How To Prepare:

1. Take a mixing bowl. Add the eggs, cream, salt and pepper and beat well and put aside.

2. Take a large skillet and heat 1 tablespoon of butter.

3. Then add the onion and spinach and stir constantly.

4. Next, pour the egg mixture and stir until everything becomes scrambled and cooked till light, fluffy and yellow.

5. Serve hot.

3. Bacon & olive omelet (Serves 4)

Fat Ingredients:

8 large free-range eggs

16 thin slices bacon

Other Ingredients:

20 pitted black olives

Pinch of pink Himalayan or sea salt

Freshly ground black pepper

How to Prepare:

1. Cut the olives into thin slices.

2. Lay the bacon, preferably free-range or organic, equally on the surface of the pan and roast for about 5 minutes.

3. Put the eggs into a mixing bowl with a pinch of salt and pepper and beat them well with a whisk or fork.

4. Turn the bacon on the other side when it gets slightly golden in color.

5. Lower the heat and pour in the eggs equally all over the pan.

6. Use a spatula to bring in the omelet from the sides towards the center for the first 30 seconds.

7. Sprinkle with sliced olives and cook for another minute or until the top appears to be almost cooked and firm.

8. Ease the omelet's edges with a spatula. Turn off the heat and serve the omelet on to a plate.

4. Keto Scrambled Eggs (Serves 4)

Fat Ingredients:

8 large eggs

1 tablespoon butter

1 cup shredded Cheddar cheese

½ cup diced sugar-free turkey or chicken ham

¼ cup heavy cream

Other Ingredients:

1 teaspoon salt

½ teaspoon black pepper

½ cup chopped onion

⅓ cup chopped red and green peppers

Chopped scallions for garnish (optional)

How to Prepare:

1. In a large mixing bowl, whisk eggs, cream, salt, and black pepper.

2. Melt the butter in a medium skillet over medium heat. Add egg mixture and stir.

3. When the eggs begin to scramble, add the ham, onion, and peppers.

4. Continue to stir until eggs are almost cooked. Add the cheddar cheese and stir.

5. Flourless Cream Cheese Pancakes (Serves 4)

Fat Ingredients:

4 eggs

4 oz. cream cheese

Other Ingredients:

1 tbsp. cinnamon

2 tbsp. coconut flour

1 packet of Stevia in the Raw

How to Prepare:

1. Combine/mix all the ingredients in a mixing bowl until smooth.

2. Heat up a non-stick pan or skillet on medium high, and coat it with butter or coconut oil.

3. Pour the batter as if it was a regular pancake batter.

4. Cook on one side most of the way before flipping.

5. Top with butter, and/or sugar-free syrup.

6. Keto Eggs Benedict (Serves 4)

Fat Ingredients:

8 large eggs

2 tablespoon butter

8 slices sugar-free Canadian bacon

2 cups Hollandaise Sauce

1 large avocado, cut into 8 pieces

How to Prepare:

1. Heat up a medium skillet over medium-high heat and add the butter. Crack eggs into the pan. Cook for 2 minutes and then flip eggs, using care not to break yolks.

2. Cook for another 2 minutes or until white is completely cooked, but yolk is still runny.

3. Transfer eggs to a plate.

4. Top each egg with a slice of Canadian bacon and a slice of avocado. Pour the sauce onto each egg.

7. High-Fat Ham, Cheese, and Egg Casserole (Serves 6)

Fat Ingredients:

12 large eggs

2 cups cooked diced cooked ham (make sure this does not contain any sugar)

½ cup shredded mozzarella cheese

½ cup shredded Cheddar cheese

Other Ingredients:

4 cups broccoli florets

½ cup chopped scallions

Bunches of broccoli (approximately one cup)

How to Prepare:

1. Preheat oven to 375°F.

2. Fill a large pot with water and bring to a boil. Blanch broccoli by putting in boiling water for 2–3 minutes.

3. Put eggs, ham, mozzarella, cheddar, and scallions in a large bowl and whisk until combined. Add broccoli.

4. Pour into a 9" × 13" baking pan and put in the oven to cook.

Lunch Recipes

1. Stuffed Avocados (Serves 4)

Fat Ingredients:

2 (6-ounce) cans tuna in oil

4 tablespoons mayonnaise

2 large avocados

Other Ingredients:

1 medium green bell pepper, chopped

1 teaspoon dried minced onion

1 teaspoon garlic salt

1 teaspoon black pepper

How to Prepare:

1. Cut avocado in half lengthwise and remove the pit. Set aside.

2. Put tuna, mayonnaise, bell pepper, dried onion, garlic, salt, and black pepper in a medium mixing bowl and mash together with a fork until combined.

3. Scoop half of the mixture into each half of the avocado.

2. Pork Tacos (Serves: 4)

Fat Ingredients:

25 oz. pork mince

½ cup of goat cheese

½ cup of mayonnaise

Other Ingredients:

3 teaspoons Taco Seasoning

4 Romaine Lettuce Leaves

How to Prepare:

1. Place the pork mince in a skillet and cook it for 20 minutes until nice and brown. Leave to cool.

2. Place the pork mince on the lettuce leaves.

3. Add the seasoning, goat cheese and a dollop of mayonnaise.

4. Wrap securely.

3. Chicken Kebabs (Serves up to 5)

Fat Ingredients:

1.5 lbs. chicken tenderloins (approx. 10)

1/2 tbsp. rosemary olive oil (or regular)

Other Ingredients:

10 6" rosemary skewers (soaked in water for at least 1 hour)

A few sprigs of fresh thyme

1/2 tbsp. garlic salt

1/2 tbsp. lemon pepper seasoning

How to Prepare:

1. Preheat oven to 350 degrees.

2. Soak the rosemary skewers for at least 1 hour in water.

3. Use a short sharp knife to twiddle a point on the end of each stick.

4. Toss chicken with ingredients. Slide the leaves off the thyme sprigs and sprinkle them in.

5. Skewer the tenderloin with a rosemary stick.

6. Bake at 350 F for 40 minutes.

4. Sausage Balls (Serves 10 – good to store)

Fat Ingredients:

2 cups of sausages shredded

½ cup of cheddar cheese

½ cup of cottage cheese

1 egg

1 tablespoon butter

Other Ingredients:

1 teaspoon of chili flakes

½ cup of red peppers

¼ teaspoon of mustard powder

How to Prepare:

1. Preheat an oven to 350 degrees.

2. Add the egg, chili, and red peppers in a bowl and mix/whisk until the ingredients are mixed completely.

3. Mix in the remaining ingredients.

4. Using a wooden baking spoon, or cookie scoop, remove the mixture, and hand-roll the sausage into about two dozen sausage balls.

5. Place the formed balls on a buttered baking pan, or cookie sheet.

6. Bake for about 15 minutes. Serve.

7. You may also store the cooked sausage bags in a covered bowl, or sandwich bags in the refrigerator for later use.

5. Tarragon Tuna (Serves 2)

Fat Ingredients:

Two 6-ounce tuna steaks, 1 inch thick

2 teaspoons mayonnaise

1 teaspoon olive oil

Other Ingredients:

2 tablespoons minced fresh or 2 teaspoons dried tarragon plus tarragon sprigs for garnish

Salt and cracked pepper to taste

How to Prepare:

1. Stir together the mayo and tarragon in a small bowl. Cover and set aside.

2. Heat a heavy skillet or ridged grill pan over medium-high heat.

3. Pat the tuna dry with paper towels, then season to taste with salt and cracked pepper. Dab olive oil over the surfaces of the fish.

4. Pan grilled the fish for about 3 minutes per side for medium. Transfer to warmed dinner plates.

5. Top each steak with a dollop of tarragon mayonnaise, and garnish with tarragon sprigs. Place a mound of squash beside the tuna.

6. Tuna and Egg Salad (Serves 2)

Fat Ingredients:

2 large hard-boiled eggs

2 (6-ounce) cans tuna (try to get those packed in oil

1⁄2 cup mayonnaise

Other Ingredients:

1⁄4 cup diced white onion

1⁄4 cup sugar-free relish

1⁄2 teaspoon salt

1⁄2 teaspoon black pepper

How to Prepare:

1. Put eggs in a medium mixing bowl and mash with a fork. Add tuna and mayonnaise and mash together until ingredients are combined.

2. Stir in onion, relish, salt, and pepper.

7. Chicken Avocado Salad (Serves 2)

Fat Ingredients:

1 (12.5-ounce) can shredded chicken breast

1⁄2 cup Homemade Mayonnaise

1 teaspoon olive oil

1 medium avocado, cubed

Other Ingredients:

2 tablespoons sliced black olives

1⁄2 teaspoon garlic salt

1⁄2 teaspoon black pepper

1⁄4 teaspoon paprika

1 teaspoon fresh lemon juice

How to Prepare:

Put all ingredients in a medium mixing bowl and mash with a fork until combined.

Dinner Recipes

1. Carb-less Pork Skewers (Serves 4)

Fat Ingredients:

2 lbs. pork shoulder

1 cup virgin olive oil (may be reused later on)

Other ingredients:

Juice from 2 large lemons

2 tbsp. balsamic vinegar

4 tbsp. freshly chopped mint

4 tbsp. freshly chopped oregano

2 tsp. sea salt

Dash of freshly ground black pepper

4 wooden or stainless steel skewers

How to Prepare:

1. To prepare the marinade, rinse the mint and oregano and drain thoroughly. Chop the herbs and preserve these apart in a small bowl.

2. Cube the pork into big cubes. Place them in a medium bowl and pour the olive oil on them.

3. Add the chopped herbs and season with balsamic vinegar. Season with salt and freshly grounded black pepper to taste.

4. Combine all the ingredients, and ensure the meat is submerged in oil. Let it relax in the fridge for 8 to 12 hours.

5. When the meat is marinated, use the grill to preheat the oven to 450 degrees. Note that the meat will barely change color after you take it out from the fridge. This is fine.

6. Skewer the meat pieces in four skewer sticks. Place them on a rack and within the oven.

7. After about 10 minutes, flip the skewers, and cook until done.

2. Sea Bass with Mango Chutney, Ginger, and Black Sesame Seeds (Makes 2 servings)

Fat Ingredients:

Two 6-ounce striped bass fillets

1 tablespoon sesame oil

Cooking spray

Other Ingredients:

1 tablespoon minced fresh ginger (see note)

1 tablespoon soy sauce

Salt and freshly milled black pepper to taste

¼ cup mango chutney

3 cups shredded iceberg lettuce

Ginger and Hot Red Pepper Vinaigrette

How to Prepare:

1. Preheat the oven to 425°F. Spray an 8 X 8 X 8-inch Pyrex baking dish with cooking spray.

2. Place the fillets in the baking dish. Sprinkle each fillet with ginger, soy sauce, and sesame oil. Lightly salt and pepper. Cover the dish with foil and bake for 10 minutes.

3. Remove from the oven and spoon 2 tablespoons of chutney onto each fillet. Return to the oven and bake, uncovered, for 5 more minutes.

4. Toss the shredded lettuce with the dressing. Divide between two plates and top each one with a fillet.

3. Roasted Butterfish (Serves 4)

Fat Ingredients:

Four giant butterfish fillets

8 tablespoon butter or ghee

Other Ingredients:

4 cloves garlic

4 teaspoons freshly chopped thyme

Pinch sea salt

Juice from 1 lemon

How to Prepare:

1. Begin by seasoning the butterfish fillets with a little bit of salt and place them on a plate.

2. Soften the butter, add the herbs and crushed garlic and blend all the pieces collectively in a small bowl.

3. Pour the butter combination over the fish.

4. Warm a non-stick pan over medium heat and add the fish.

5. Roast for about 2 to 3 minutes on both sides until cooked and the fish will get a crispy golden texture. Be certain that the fillet is totally cooked by slicing into it. Cooked flesh will look opaque.

6. Place the fish onto a serving plate and squeeze a little bit of lemon over it. Serve sizzling.

4. Broccoli and Ham Quiche (Serves 12)

Fat Ingredients:

10 large organic eggs or 12 medium eggs

2 cups of thinly sliced ham

1 cup of grated cheddar cheese

1 ½ cups of heavy cream

3 tablespoons of olive oil

Other Ingredients:

12 cups of cubed broccoli flowerets

2 teaspoons of chili flakes

How to Prepare:

1. Preheat the oven to 350F.

2. Take 2 deep 10-inch quiche pans. Grease them with a bit of olive oil and keep aside.

3. Take a large mixing bowl. Crack all the eggs and pour into the bowl. Then add the heavy cream, chili flakes, and beat well until it has all been mixed well.

4. Take each quiche pan and place the ham slices and broccoli flowerets evenly in each pan. Then sprinkle the cheese over them and finally pour the egg and cream mixture over it.

5. Bake for 20 minutes until the top is golden brown in color. Prick with a fork till the bottom of quiche to check if done. If it is clean, then the quiche is ready to enjoy.

5. Baked Salmon (Serves 4)

Fat Ingredients:

4 6-ounce salmon fillets

3 tbsp. olive oil

Other Ingredients:

2 tablespoons of lemon juice

1 tablespoon each of minced parsley, mint, garlic, paprika, sunflower seeds (slightly crushed)

How to Prepare:

1. Clean the fillet and put aside.

2. Place all the other ingredients in another bowl, and mix well and pour onto the fish. Marinate the fillet for 6 hours.

3. After 6 hours, place in a baking dish and bake for 1 hour at 250F until flaky and cooked.

4. Serve with sour cream, green beans and apricots.

6. Fried Chicken (Serves 4)

Fat Ingredients:

1 pound or 4 (4-ounce) boneless, skinless chicken breasts

1/2 cup crushed pork rinds

1/2 cup grated Parmesan cheese

2 large eggs

2 tablespoons coconut oil

Other Ingredients:

1/2 teaspoon garlic powder

1/4 teaspoon onion powder

1/4 teaspoon dried minced onion

1/4 teaspoon salt

1/4 teaspoon black pepper

How to Prepare:

1. Put pork rinds, Parmesan cheese, garlic powder, onion powder, minced onion, salt, and black pepper in a large mixing bowl and stir until well mixed.

2. Crack eggs into a separate bowl and whisk.

3. Dip each chicken breast into eggs and then coat in pork rind mixture, making sure the chicken is completely covered.

4. Heat coconut oil in a skillet over medium-high heat. Place the chicken breasts into the pan. Let them cook for 5–7 minutes or until pork rind crust is browned. Flip chicken over and let them cook for another 5–7 minutes until cooked through.

5. Serve hot.

7. One Pan Baked Chicken Thighs (Serves 2)

Fat Ingredients:

4 chicken thighs (deboned, skin on)

1/4 cup olive oil

Other Ingredients:

2 zucchinis

1/2 cup carrot (sliced)

2 tablespoons balsamic vinegar

1 cup daikon radish

1-inch length of cube ginger, minced

How to Prepare:

1. Pre-heat an oven to 350 degrees.

2. Use a paper towel, and pat the chicken thighs dry.

3. Wrap the skins around the chicken thighs, and place these on a buttered or greased baking sheet.

4. Slice the radish and zucchinis, and with the carrots, place them around the thigh pieces.

5. Using a small bowl mix the vinegar, oil, and ginger – this is your sauce. Pour the mix over the chicken.

5. Season with salt and pepper and bake the chicken thighs for 30 minutes.

Conclusion

I hope this book was able to help you to achieve not only your weight loss goals, but to have a more vibrant, healthier lifestyle beyond losing weight and looking great.

The next step in your journey is to start listing down your weight goals, changing your food shopping lists, and prepare for a new and sexier wardrobe!

Finally, if you enjoyed this book, then I'd like to ask you for a favor, would you be kind enough to leave a review for this book on Amazon? It'd be greatly appreciated!

Thank you and good luck!

REFERENCES

Introduction

1. Brown, H. (2015). Planning to Go on a Diet? One Word of Advice: Don't. Retrieved December 30, 2016, from http://www.slate.com/articles/health_and_science/medical_examiner/2015/03/diets_do_not_work_the_thin_evidence_that_losing_weight_makes_you_healthier.html

2. Average woman spends 31 years on a diet, researchers say. (2007). Retrieved December 30, 2016, from http://www.dailymail.co.uk/health/article-430913/Average-woman-spends-31-years-diet-researchers-say.html

Chapter 1. The False Promises of Carbohydrates

1. Office of Dietary Supplements - Daily Values (DVs). (n.d.). Retrieved December 18, 2016, from https://ods.od.nih.gov/HealthInformation/dailyvalues.aspx 2. USDA "Plate"

2. Choose MyPlate. (n.d.). Retrieved December 25, 2016, from https://www.choosemyplate.gov/

3. Longevity/Health in Ancient Paleolithic vs Neolithic Peoples. (n.d.). Retrieved December 20, 2016, from http://www.beyondveg.com/nicholson-w/angel-1984/angel-1984-1a.shtml

4. DeWitte, S. N., & Bekvalac, J. (2010). Oral Health and Frailty in the Medieval English Cemetery of St. Mary Graces. Retrieved December 22, 2016, from https://www.ncbi.nlm.nih.gov/pmc/articles/PMC3094918/

5. A Brief History of Heart Disease. (n.d.). Retrieved December 22, 2016, from http://forum.prisonplanet.com/index.php?topic=206436.0

Chapter 2. The Chemistry of Eating

1. McDonald, L., & McDonald, L. (1998). The ketogenic diet: a complete guide for the dieter and practitioner. Austin, TX: The Author.

2. Metabolic processes (2010). Retrieved December 26, 2016, from https://www.youtube.com/watch?v=mtHDjC1emGs

3. Overview Metabolism. (n.d.). Retrieved December 24, 2016, from http://chemistry.elmhurst.edu/vchembook/600glycolysis.html

Chapter 3. How We Get Fat And Sick From Food

1. Cordain, L. (2011). The Paleo diet: lose weight and get healthy by eating the foods you were designed to eat. Hoboken, NJ: Wiley.

Chapter 4. Ketosis And Ketogenesis

1. Boyers, Lindsay (2015). The everything guide to the ketogenic diet: a step-by-step guide to the ultimate fat-burning diet plan! Avon, MA: Adams Media.

2. Ray, N. (2013). Atkins diet: complete Atkins diet guide to losing weight and feeling amazing! North Charleston, SC: Createspace.

Chapter 5. Ketogenic Diet Basics

1. Excellent carb-counting resource include:

http://www.carb-counter.net/

2. There are a great multitude of apps for both Android and IOS. Listed below is a tiny sample of what's available:

Calorie, Carb & Fat Counter by Virtuagym

Calorie Counter by My Fitness Pal

Low Carb Foods Guide by deluxapps

3. Boyers, Lindsay (2015). The everything guide to the ketogenic diet: a step-by-step guide to the ultimate fat-burning diet plan! Avon, MA: Adams Media.

4. (2016). Retrieved December 26, 2016, from https://www.youtube.com/watch?v=H7mjm9LyW-c

Chapter 6. What to Eat. And What Not To!

1. H. (2016). Complete Keto Diet Food List: What to Eat and Avoid | The KetoDiet Blog. Retrieved December 24, 2016, from

http://ketodietapp.com/Blog/post/2015/01/03/Keto-Diet-Food-List-What-to-Eat-and-Avoid

2, Johnson, R. A., Says, R., Says, J. R., Says, C., Says, L., Says, L., . . . Says, A. (2016). The Ultimate Ketogenic Diet Food List (What to Eat on The Keto Diet). Retrieved December 22, 2016, from https://dietingwell.com/ketogenic-diet-food-list/

3. H. (2016). Ketogenic Diet Food List - What Are Keto Foods? (PDF Download). Retrieved December 20, 2016, from http://paleomagazine.com/ketogenic-diet-food-list

Chapter 7. Do's and Don't's

1. H. (2016). How To Low Carb: 15 Common Weight Loss Mistakes | The KetoDiet Blog. Retrieved December 27, 2016, from http://ketodietapp.com/Blog/post/2016/01/11/how-to-low-carb-15-common-weight-loss-mistakes

2. 13 common keto mistakes. (2016). Retrieved December 22, 2016, from https://www.ketovangelist.com/13-common-keto-mistakes/

Chapter 8. Happy Keto Eating Recipes

1. Slajerova, M. (2016). Sweet & savory fat bombs: 100 delicious treats for fat fasts, ketogenic, paleo, and low-carb diets. Beverly, MA: Fair Winds.

2. The Best Keto Recipes. (n.d.). Retrieved December 23, 2016, from https://www.dietdoctor.com/low-carb/recipes/best-keto-recipes

3. Low Carb Recipes for Ketogenic Diets. (n.d.). Retrieved December 27, 2016, from http://www.ketogenic-diet-resource.com/low-carb-recipes.html

Atkins Diet

The Ultimate Guide to Atkins Diet

Introduction

I want to thank you and congratulate you for downloading *Atkins: Ultimate Guide to Atkins!*

Weight loss is something that nearly everyone struggles with, especially as we get older. As our metabolism slows down, it is much easier to gain fat, lose muscle, and face new health ailments that keep us from enjoying life. If you do a simple google search about how to lose weight, thousands of articles, diet plans, and workout routines will immediately pop up. Of course, the general idea for any weight loss plan is to eat right and exercise, right? So, out of the hundreds of methods you can choose from, which one is right for you?

Atkins has been proven to be the most efficient and effective weight loss plan out there. It has helped millions of people around the globe find health and happiness through its strict but effective regiment. The question is, how do you know if Atkins will work for you and give you the results you want? The answer is simple. Atkins works for everyone whose goal is to burn fat and become healthier. This method in particular works because it keeps you from consuming foods that have any form of sugar, so that your body burns pure fat for energy instead.

The modern diet is largely made up of carbohydrates and fats, which do not work well together and contribute to the development of several diseases. This guide will teach you everything you need to know about the Atkins diet, as well as how your body functions using basic macronutrients. Through carefully laid out steps and strategies, you will learn how to become truly independent from sugar addiction, cravings, and common factors that attribute to falling off the wagon and going back to your old eating habits.

Here is an inescapable fact: most people will fail in their weight loss attempts. More than sixty- percent of the people who create goals and want to become healthier are unsuccessful and stay unhappy with their bodies. This guide gives you all the information you could possibly need to not only be successful in your journey of losing weight, but also become an inspiration and role model for other individuals who aspire to greater health. Knowledge is your greatest advantage to any new goal, and this book will teach you the science behind the Atkins diet, how cutting out carbohydrates can save your life, and a complete twenty – one-day meal plan to get you through the first phase of the program.

If you do not develop your understanding of weight loss, you will spend years looking for "the secret" or "magic supplement" that doesn't exist. Too many people look for the easiest way to get what they want, without acknowledging that the greatest success comes from a little struggle and a lot of willpower. Atkins is not just a dieting program, but the most trusted and effective strategy to burning fat and achieving your goals that you will ever find.

It's time for you to become an amazing and happier you. Think of all the things you will miss out on if you do not change your habits and lead a healthier life. Now is the time to take control of your lifestyle and change for the better. You *can* be skinner, toned, strong, and healthy; if you choose to be. It is time for you to begin your journey of transformation and rejuvenation. Good luck and enjoy!

Chapter 1: What is Atkins? The Game- Changing Weight Loss Plan

The theory of dieting has been around for as long as society has wanted a solution to their weight loss and health needs. There are dozens of cultures, religions, and countries around the world who all promote and live by different eating habits; all of which have their own benefits and disadvantages. The various lifestyles lead to the cultivation of hundreds of diet plans and programs that all promise to help you lose weight. An idea that was not often practiced in the twentieth century is now a multi- billion- dollar institution that promotes and feeds off of the public's insecurities and resolutions. However, it was not until recently that any of these methods were particularly effective.

We live in an age where food is accessible and cheap, which makes it easy to over eat and make poor choices with meals. Many diets share the same focus of cutting out calories, so that your body begins utilizing more calories than what you are intaking to create energy. This leads to less water weight and overall loss of fat, muscle, and water. The general foundation of this method works, but not to the fullest extent of what you truly want when changing your eating habits so drastically. Eating in a caloric deficit will allow you to lose weight, but it will not help you to keep the weight off for good. In fact, many diets often leave the participant hungry and craving sugar- loaded foods. After your body is starved of calories for so long, the individual experiences a great relapse and binges more than they have in the past. This leads to gaining back all of the weight that you just lost, and then some. The vicious cycle continues as another weight loss program is found and the individual picks up right where they initially began. Different diet, same concept.

The reality is that even though most diets are based off of cutting out calories, there is not much evidence that suggests doing so will manifest long- term success. Thus, the search for a diet that works on a different strategy for overall health and weight loss continues. This is where Atkins comes into play. What many have considered to be another fad diet, has brought success in the journey for long- term weight loss for anyone who has dared to take on the challenge of cutting out something other than calories from their diet. Atkins takes a more scientific approach to the theory of losing weight by analyzing how the modernized western diet has changed.

Today, we consume more carbohydrates than ever before and rely on bread and starch as staples for every meal. Cereal, pasta, and bread on consumed on a daily basis, which leads to the body storing more fat and living off the short bursts of energy that simple carbohydrates fuel. There is much to be said about how carbs and fats interact with your body's chemistry; however, that will be discussed in a later chapter.

The Atkins diet was made famous by physician Dr. Robert C. Atkins through is best- selling book that explained the diet in 1972. Since the release of his work, the Atkins diet has reached all four corners of the globe and inspired millions of people to look at weight loss with a different perspective. Many books and articles have reanalyzed and digested the diet time and time again, all with their own unique take on the matter. At first, the Atkins diet was deemed unhealthy and even confronted mainstream health authorities for their use of carbohydrates and saturated fat. However, there have been dozens of studies that have proven the many benefits that Atkins has to offer, despite what skeptics and critics may believe.

Atkins does not promote the idea of cutting out calories from your diet, but simple carbohydrates and sugar. This idea was entirely new, but proved successful for many. This is because when you reduce your carb intake and increase your protein intake, your appetite greatly subsides and end up consuming less calories without even realizing it. Diets that are high in carbohydrates leave your appetite satisfied for a short amount of time, as cravings and hunger pangs will ensue just an hour after eating. Atkins begins by completely cutting out carbs, and then slowly reintroducing complex carbohydrates once your body has learned how to run efficiently without unnecessary sugar. There are several rules and guidelines that are outlined throughout the diet, however the complete long- term alteration of one's eating habits encourages individuals view Atkins as a lifestyle change, rather than a short- term solution to losing weight.

The key to staying successful with Atkins is sticking to it, even after the first phase is over. You will experience cravings and even perhaps lapses of judgement, just like you would have with any other dieting program. However, Atkins does not encourage you to keep to a restrictive regiment for too long, and reintroduces foods that you love as you learn how to correctly consume them in relation to the high consumption of protein and fat that Atkins requires. Now, you may be wondering how you could possibly give up bread and other sugary foods that have become staples to your diet. Once you have completed the first phase of the program, you will crave those foods less and be able to enjoy small amounts later on as you progress through the program.

Atkins Phases Broken Down

Phase 1:

Phase one is designed to help your body detox from sugar and become reliant on protein and fat for energy instead of carbohydrates. During this stage, you will consume under twenty grams of carbohydrates each day for approximately two weeks. Throughout the extent of phase one, you will eat meals that are high in fat, protein, and count your carbs through vegetables, like leafy greens.

Phase one allows your metabolism to kick- start into weight loss mode. So, that you can reprogram the way your body utilizes macronutrients. This first part of the programs is often mistaken for the structure of the entire program, but this is an inaccurate judgement. While you function off just twenty carbs a day, you begin understand the maximum grams of net carbs that you can eat while also experiencing weight loss and adequate energy levels. This is referred to as your personal carb balance, which will be established as you continue into the next phase.

This phase should last for a minimum of two weeks, although you can safely follow the guidelines of this phase for as long as you need to if your goal is to lose as much weight as possible in the shortest amount of time. In this case, you will continue with phase one until you are fifteen pounds away from your target weight.

Phase 2:

Once you have achieved your goal weight with phase one, it is time to begin phase two. During this part of the diet plan, the participant will slowly start to add in new types of carbohydrates. The purpose is to correctly reintroduce the right kind of carbohydrates into your meal plan, so that you are still giving your body the nutrients it needs while still losing weight. You will begin eating nuts, low- carb veggies, and small amounts of fruit; and you will continue this phase until you are within ten pounds of your target weight.

Keep in mind that just because you can start eating carbs again does not mean that you can eat whatever you want, as long as it isn't too much. Nuts, strawberries, melon, seeds, cottage cheese, blueberries, and cottage cheese are a few examples of what you are limited to during phase two. The purpose of adding some more carbohydrates to your meal in this phase is to help you keep your momentum that you gained in the beginning of phase one, while still attempting to find your personal carbohydrate balance. Although you may stay dedicated to phase two until you are within ten pounds of your target weight, you can transition into phase three sooner if you are willing to let your weight loss pace slow a little.

Phase 3:

Phase three marks the progress that you have made, as you are closer than ever to your target weight. At this point in the Atkins plan, you will add even more carbohydrates into your diet until your weight loss slightly slows down. This phase is meant to help you fine- tune your diet so that you can eventually focus on maintaining your weight loss when you come into phase four. During phase three, you will see how much you can increase your daily net carb consumption while still maintaining weight loss during while reintroducing a wider variety of carbohydrate- filled foods. You will remain in phase three until you have achieved your goal weight and maintained it for at least thirty days.

Phase 4:

Phase four is designed to help you maintain your weight loss and new health diet. During this part of the Atkins plan, you are allowed to consume as many health carbohydrates as your body can take without paying close attention to your weight. This phase is regarded as a lifetime lifestyle, when you generally stick with the meal plan as a long- term commitment; eating the same foods that you have already been consuming with each new phase. Some foods that you may have tried to reintroduce earlier on, your body can now adequately handle. As long as you maintain your target weight, you can continue experimenting with small amounts of different carbs and other foods that you enjoy.

The phases that mark the progression of the Atkin diet may seem a bit complicated or even unnecessary. However, the entire program is designed to help your body overcome the addiction to carbohydrates while still enjoying the tasty foods that you love. The truth of the matter is that you are the only one who fully understands how your body works. You will notice right away if part of the meal plan does not work for you and your needs, and can easily alter your strategy accordingly. While giving up carbohydrates for any length of time can prove to be challenging, the first phase only lasts for two weeks and the benefits of detoxing from sugar can last a lifetime.

Chapter 2: The Basics of Atkins

Efficient protein intake and working your body into a ketogenic state are critical components to maximizing fat loss and maintaining muscle during the Atkins diet. While the first phase of Atkins may require a minimum of two weeks of dedication, it will take approximately three weeks for your body to become adapted to its natural ketogenic function. During the beginning phase of Atkins, nitrogen loss may occur if your carb consumption is extremely low. This is due to the fact that when your carb intake decreases, your body resorts to converting protein into glucose. Approximately sixteen percent of protein is nitrogen, and thus the loss of muscle occurs and your metabolic rate will decrease. Issues like this arise when you are not consuming adequate amounts of protein. Although your body is used to converting carbohydrates into glucose for energy, it can efficiently do this with protein and fats as well. The reason that our bodies do not already default to this way of functioning is because the modern diet is largely made up of carbohydrates and sugary foods; which are easier to break down into glucose.

This issue is especially inconvenient for body builders and other gym goers, as building muscle is essential for their regiment. So, how many carbohydrates do you need in order to maintain muscle and spare protein loss? The greatest challenge that comes with limiting your carb intake is that your body can go into starvation mode for too long, which leads to muscle loss. Starvation mode occurs when you consume less than fifteen carbs per day; this is necessary for your body to utilize its fat stores for energy. When you increase your carb consumption to fifty grams per day, your body is less dependent on amino acids for glycogenesis. Glycogenesis occurs through two different mechanisms. Firstly, when the increased carb consumption results in high blood glucose and insulin levels, which restricts your cortisol release. And secondly, when the carbs supply the brain with glucose, inhibiting the breakdown of protein in the body.

While keeping to the Atkins diet, your overall protein intake should account for at least seventy – percent of your diet; with your fat intake making up twenty – percent, and carbohydrates accounting for the remaining ten percent. As you move into the second phase, your carb intake will increase by ten percent, as your fat and protein intake decrease slightly. As you continue through the program, you will slowly alter the percentage of your macronutrient intake as your body adjusts to the new meal plan.

You can easily figure out how many grams of protein, fat, and carbohydrates you should consume with each meal and on a daily basis by using online macronutrient calculators. The website will ask a variety of questions based on your goals and physical health in order to determine the correct macro proportions for your diet. You will have to fill in information regarding your:

- Age

- Weight
- Sex
- Height
- Daily or Weekly Activity Level
  - Sedentary
  - Lightly Active
  - Moderately Active
  - Very Active
- The Kind of Exercise You Typically Perform
- Current Body Fat Percentage
- Main Objective Regarding Your Diet
  - Lose Weight
  - Maintain Weight
  - Gain Muscle

What to Eat on the Atkins Diet?

Meat

- Bacon
- Beef
- Fish/ Seafood
- Poultry
- Pork
- Turkey

Eggs

Vegetables

- Artichokes
- Asparagus

- Broccoli
- Cabbage
- Celery
- Cauliflower
- Kale
- Lettuce
- Mushroom
- Onions
- Peppers
- Radishes
- Spinach
- Spaghetti Squash
- Zucchini

Fats/Oils

- Coconut
- Flaxseed
- Olive
- Sesame
- Sunflower

Dairy

- Butter
- Cheese
- Full Fat Cream Cheese
- Full Fat Yogurt
- Heavy Whipping Cream
- Sour Cream

Nuts and Seeds

(All nuts are permitted during Phases 2-4)

Seeds:

- Chia
- Flax
- Pumpkin
- Sesame
- Sunflower

Drinks

- Water
- Tea (Black)
- Coffee (Black)

Foods to Avoid While on the Atkins Diet

Breads and Grains

- Bagels
- Barley
- Couscous
- English Muffins
- Kaiser Rolls
- Oats
- Pasta
- Rice
- Tortillas
- Products Containing Flour
- Whole Grains

Vegetables (During Phase One Only)

- Beans
- Carrots
- Chickpeas

- Corn
- Hummus
- Lentils
- Peas
- Potatoes
- Soy Beans
- Tomatoes
- Turnips

Sweets

- Cake
- Cookies
- Ice Cream
- Pastries
- Pies
- Pudding
- Gelatin

Sugars and Sweeteners

- White Sugar
- Brown Sugar
- Sucralose
- Aspartame
- Erythritol
- Agave Nectar
- Xylitol

Drinks

- Alcohol
- Energy Drinks
- Hot Chocolate
- Juice

- Milk
- Protein Shakes
- Soft Drinks
- Sports Drinks
- Sweetened Teas

Vegetable Oils and Fats

- Canola Oil
- Vegetable Oil
- Soybean Oil
- Trans Fats

High – Carb Fruits

- Apples
- Bananas
- Grapes
- Oranges
- Pears

Adding Carbs Back into Your Diet After Phase One

Despite what many people may believe, the Atkins program is relatively flexible. The most difficult part of beginning this diet is the first phase, in which you will minimize your carb intake. Once the induction phase is over, you are allowed to slowly integrate healthy carbohydrates back into your diet. This includes vegetables that are higher in carbohydrates, fruits, starches, and healthy grains such as oats and brown rice. However, once you have made it to the final phase of the program, you will need to maintain that lifestyle for the long haul; even if you have achieved your weight loss and health goals.

It is crucial that you keep to the diet you have formed during the final phase because your body will react differently to the old foods that you used to eat. You may have bloating and trouble digesting as your body becomes sensitive to certain foods that may be difficult for it to process. Regardless, even if your body does not have a negative reaction to high carbohydrate food products, you will gain back the weight you lose during the last three phases. Of course, this rings true for any weight loss program you try.

Atkins allows you to eat the delicious foods you love, such as bacon and cheese. However, as you begin introducing new foods during the second phase, you can experiment with different types of carbohydrates. As your net carb intake increases to fifty grams, you can start eating dark chocolate, fruits, oats, etc. One of the most difficult factors for many people on this diet is finding foods to snack on. While you may not be able to go to your default bag of potato chips or candy, there are plenty of options to keep you satisfied with your salty and sweet cravings. Some examples of low – carb snacks include:

- Hard – boiled eggs
- Cheese
- Nuts and seeds
- Yogurt
- Berries and whipped cream
- Green tea

Chapter 3: The Science Behind the Diet: Why it Works

We have been lead to believe that the more carbs and less fat we have in our diets, the healthier we will be. After all, carbohydrates are a source of energy, while fat makes us fat. Right? Actually, this way of thinking is completely wrong. Our bodies are capable of many things, and one of them is converting fat and protein into energy. Why would you want to completely change your diet just so your body uses fat for energy? Because fat does not make you fat: sugar does. In fact, carbohydrates are made up of starch, fiber, and sugar. When broken down during the digestive process, the majority of these nutrients are stored away for later as fat. This means that the more carbohydrates you eat, the more your body will store away for later, as it only takes a small number of carbs to function on a day to day basis.

Fat, on the other hand, does not get stored away as fat cells when you consume too much of it; and neither does protein. When you cut out carbs from your diet and increase the amount of protein and fat you eat, the way your body functions entirely changes. Its traditional energy source is no longer available, so it must resort to using other nutrients for energy. When this happens, your body begins using your stored fat as fuel, and you begin to lose weight. This process is called ketosis.

Ketosis is something that your body does every day, whether you eat carbs or not. However, eating a low carb, high fat diet gives this process a natural boost. Your body breaks carbohydrates down into glucose, because glucose is needed to create energy. When your body does not have glucose to process, it goes into a deep state of ketosis. Your body will burn fat stores, creating molecules: ketones. Ketones occur when your body breaks down fat into fatty acids in the liver during a process known as beta- oxidation. Although during the first few weeks of ketosis, the individual will experience energy lulls, studies have shown that your body runs up to seventy percent more efficiently than when it uses glucose for energy. This coincides perfectly with our evolution as human beings. Our ancestors did not have access to the food that we eat today, and therefore relied on protein and fat to keep them nourished.

While your body is in ketosis, it is possible that it produces too many ketone bodies. Therefore, the body with naturally expel of excess ketones through urine. However, this is not a sign that your state of ketosis is slowing down, but that your brains has enough BHB (beta- hydroxybutyric acid) to keep functioning at a higher level. Although the idea of burning pure fat sounds great, your body does need glucose to maintain maximum health, which is why phase one is the only time during Atkins when you will severely limit your carb intake.

Your body can theoretically completely become independent from carbohydrates. This is due to the breakdown of excess protein in your diet. Protein can be used for energy, building muscle, and keeping your bones strong. However, when you eat too much protein, approximately fifty- six percent will be turned into glucose in the bloodstream. Therefore, it is crucial that you keep a strict eye on your protein intake during the first three phases; so you don't accidently knock your body out of ketosis.

It is important to recognize that ketosis and starvation are two entirely different things. Starvation occurs when your body has no source of food or nutrition. This will result in muscle loss as your body begins using its own stores of protein in your muscles to stay alive. Ketosis is a temporary state of fasting that will encourage your body to use some of your fat stores for energy to induce weight loss. When done correctly, the ketogenic process will preserve your muscle tissue.

What to Expect During Phase One: Introducing Your Body to Ketosis

When you start any diet, you will notice weight loss almost immediately. However, this "weight loss" is not stored fat, but simply water weight. The human body is mostly made up of water. When you consume a lot of carbohydrates, you may experience bloating, even the day after consuming a big meal. This is because carbohydrate molecules and water molecules cling to each other, resulting in excess water weight. During the beginning of the Atkins diet, you will first drop any bloating that is caused by retaining water.

Once your body has dropped its water weight, you will start to lose real pounds of fat. Although it is easy to get hung up on the scale, it is more important to note the more obvious physical changes. While you may only drop a few pounds when you weigh in, your waist may have shrunk by a few inches. Lost inches are relatively more significant than numbers on a scale. Your clothes will feel a bit looser even if the number on the scale does not budge. During the Atkins program, is it normal for your body to fluctuate on a daily basis. Keeping a constant eye on the scale is not an efficient way of measuring your progress on this diet.

Carbohydrate- filled foods often contain massive amounts of sodium, which is not necessarily a bad thing. As your body flushes out toxins, ketones, and other excess nutrients, it will begin to lose electrolytes as well. If you begin feeling ill or a lack of energy, try drinking full sodium broth every day. This technique will also stop constipation, headaches, and muscle cramps during the first phase.

The best way to begin the Atkins program is to lose any expectations you may have. Everyone's body is different, and will react in different ways to the sudden change in diet. Your friend may have lost seven pounds within the first week of phase one, but there is no way of knowing if you will lose the same amount. Just know that during induction, you are cleansing your body in the most efficient way, and becoming a better and healthier you with each passing day.

Chapter 4: Top Benefits of Cutting and Limiting Carbohydrates

Low carb- high fat diets have been used for thousands of years for its various healing benefits. Nearly every culture in the world recognizes some form of this program as a way to cure diseases, improve overall health, and enhance the body's natural functions. While weight loss may be your primary reason for switching to a ketogenic diet, there are other benefits that you should consider while making this transition.

1. Inhibiting Your Appetite (In a Positive Way)

Hunger is not only eventually leads to bingeing, but it is also possibly the worst side effect of dieting. Hunger is typically the main reason most people feel terrible while dieting and end up giving up on losing weight all together. Let's face it, no one likes hunger pangs. Possibly the best part about switching to a low-carb diet is the automatic reduction of your appetite. Various studies have shown that when cutting down carbs and increasing protein and fat intake, people end up eating much fewer calories than normal. Without even trying, you will already eat less than usual.

2. More Weight Loss Than You Expect

It is no secret that cutting out carbohydrates is the simplest and by far most effective method of losing weight. After learning the biological process of burning fat on the Atkins diet, it is easy to see that people on low- carb diets tend to lose more weight quicker than individuals who stick to a low- fat meal plan. Even when others may restrict calories, people who adopt a ketogenic diet will still have more success.

This is due, firstly, to the quick explement of excess water weight from the body. Additionally, due to lower insulin levels, your kidneys will also get rid of extra sodium through urination, resulting in even more weight loss. When comparing studies, experts have found that individuals who keep to a low carb diet will lose up to three times as much weight, without experiencing hunger.

The most successful weight loss stories featuring low- carb diets report sticking to the diet for longer than six months. This is because many people tend to resort back to their old eating habits after reaching their goal weight. This is why sticking with a low – carb diet as your lifestyle will create better results, as long-term commitment soon becomes second nature.

3. Most of the Fat Loss Achieved in from the Abdominal Cavity

Even though we all would love to lose fat from everywhere on our bodies, the reality is that not all fat in your body is the same. Where your fat is stored dictates how your health is affected and whether or not you are at risk for disease. Your body contains two kinds of fat: subcutaneous and visceral. Subcutaneous fat is the layer underneath your skin, while visceral fat resides in your abdominal cavity and around your organs. Too much visceral fat results in increased inflammation, insulin resistance, and metabolic dysfunction disorder; commonly found in Westernized countries.

Low- carb lifestyles are extremely effective at decreasing excess fat around your abdomen, so that stubborn belly fat is more likely to disappear during the first few phases of Atkins. The reduction of visceral fat will also reduce your potential of developing heart disease and type 2 diabetes.

4. Your Triglyceride Levels Will Drastically Decrease

Triglycerides are fat molecules. An excess of triglycerides is when there is high level of fat is in your blood stream. Elevated triglyceride levels may result in the hardening of your arteries or the development of pancreatitis. It will also dramatically increase your risk of heart attack, heart disease, and stroke. It has become common knowledge in the medical world that fasting triglycerides (how much of them are in your blood after fasting overnight) is a strong indication of potential heart disease.

While many people believe that eating a lot of fat will result in elevated triglycerides, it is really carbohydrates that are the culprit; especially in the form of simple sugar. Cutting carbs results in the dramatic decrease of blood triglycerides, which is the exact opposite result of low- fat diets.

5. Improved Levels of HDL Cholesterol

Not many people know that cholesterol comes in two forms: LDL and HDL. HDL, high density lipoprotein, is known as the "good" cholesterol. LDL and HDL direct the lipoproteins that transport cholesterol through the bloodstream. LDL actually transports the cholesterol from the liver to the rest of your body, but HDL carries it away from the rest of the body towards the liver to be reused or disposed of. The more elevated your HDL cholesterol levels are, your risk of heart disease is drastically lowered. The most efficient method of improving your HDL cholesterol levels is eating a low- carb, high- fat diet. HDL levels may only increase moderately or even go down when consuming a low- fat diet.

6. Decreased Blood Sugar Levels and Insulin Levels: In Relation to Individuals with Type 2 Diabetes

Type 2 diabetes is somewhat of an epidemic this day and age: the rising child obesity rates and poor eating habits of adults has resulted in an increase of this condition throughout the population. When we consume carbohydrates, the molecules are broken down into simple sugars, like glucose), within the digestive tract. Once broken down, the glucose enters the bloodstream and results in elevated blood sugar levels. However, high blood sugar levels are extremely toxic. Therefore, your body responds by producing the hormone insulin. Insulin communicates to your cells that there is too much glucose and they need to bring it down by either burning it or storing it.

Individuals who are health have a quick insulin response, which minimizes the blood sugar spike to prevent too much glucose from harming our bodies. However, millions of people suffer from major problems with responding to glucose spikes. Those with type 2 diabetes suffer from insulin resistance; when their cells do not recognize the insulin and therefore have a more difficult time lowering the blood sugar levels using your cells. It is crucial that your body produces enough insulin after meals to quickly lower your blood sugar; so patients with type 2 diabetes will inject even more insulin into their bodies after eating.

Cutting out carbohydrates improve your body's response to glucose spikes by eliminating the need for so much insulin. Therefore, both blood sugars and insulin dramatically decrease. In fact, keeping to a strict low/ no- carb diet will cure type 2 diabetes altogether within just a few months. However, if you are taking blood sugar- lowering medication, you should consult your doctor before making changes to your diet in order to prevent hypoglycemia (dangerously low blood sugar.

7. Your Blood Pressure Will Go Way Down

Hypertension, or elevated blood pressure, is not only a symptom of many diseases, but also a risk factor for developing new conditions. Such ailments include heart disease, heart attack, stroke, thyroid issues, diabetes, kidney disease, kidney failure, and many other diseases. Low carb diets are one of the most effective methods of quickly reducing blood pressure, which will help decrease the risk of disease and help you live a long and happy life.

8. Extremely Effective for Treating and Curing Metabolic Syndrome

Metabolic syndrome is a condition that includes a variety of serious and even fatal symptoms, including:

- Obesity

- High blood pressure

- Elevated blood sugar levels

- Elevated triglyceride levels

- Low DLD cholesterol levels

Metabolic syndrome increases the individual's risk of stroke, heart attack, heart disease, and type two diabetes. However, all symptoms of metabolic syndrome improve drastically while on a low- carb, high- fat diet. Unfortunately, major health organizations continue recommending a low- fat diet for individuals with this condition, even though it does not address the fundamental metabolic issue that causes these serious symptoms.

9. Increasingly Improves the Function of LDL Cholesterol

Low Density Lipoprotein (LDL) is known as the "bad" cholesterol and counter opposite of HDL. This is due to the fact that individuals with higher LDL levels are more likely to suffer from a heart attack. Although this idea goes against what we have been lead to believe about LDL, scientists have found that LDL matters when it comes to our health; not all LDL proteins are equal. This means that the size of the LDL protein particles is important and plays a large role in the state of your health. Individuals whose LDL is mostly made up of small particles have a heightened risk of heart disease, while people with large particles have a lower risk.

It has been found that low- carbohydrate, high- fat diets increase the size of the LDL particles, as well as reduce the number of LDL particles that are flowing through the bloodstream.

10. Low- Carbohydrate Lifestyles Help to Improve Several Brain Disorders

While low- carb diets are beneficial for a number of serious diseases, one of the most valuable uses of sticking to a ketogenic diet is acting as a therapeutic factor for life- altering brain disorders. Glucose is necessary for the brain, however only some parts of the brain are able to burn glucose. This is why your liver will create glucose out of excess protein if you stop consuming carbohydrates. However, a large part of the brain can also utilize ketones; which, as you know, are created when your body's carb consumption is very limited. This amazing and natural function of the ketogenic diet has been practiced for decades to help treat children with epilepsy when medicinal treatment fails.

In a number of cases, the Atkins diet has even cured children of epilepsy. One study concluded that more than half of the children who were fed a low- carb diet had a more than fifty percent reduction in their seizure episodes, with sixteen percent of the kids being cured altogether. The success with the low- carb, high-fat diet in epilepsy patients has inspired doctors and researchers to study the relationship between a ketogenic diet and several other disorders; for example, Parkinson's disease and Alzheimer's disease.

Part 2:

Atkins
21- Day Meal Plan

Chapter 5: 10 No- Carb Breakfast Recipes

1. Bacon, Cheese, and Avocado Breakfast Fiesta

Ingredients

½ of a Medium- Sized Tomato

1 Oz. Water

1 Medium- Sized Spring Onion

1 Slices of Cooked Bacon

1/3 Cup of Shredded Monterey Jack Cheese

½ Small Jalapeno Pepper

2 tsp. of Butter

1 tsp. of Lime Juice

½ Avocado, sliced

½ tsp. of Cilantro

2 Large Eggs

Directions:

1. Start by preparing your homemade salsa. First, chop the tomatoes, spring onion, and jalapeno pepper.

2. Combine these ingredients in bowl with the cilantro and juice from the lime. Set aside for later.

3. In a separate bowl, beat eggs with water. Then, crumble the cooked bacon and set aside.

4. Liquefy the butter at medium heat in a pan. When the pan is coated with the butter, add in half of the egg mixture. Tilt the pan so that the bottom is evenly coated with the egg, then continue cooking until the egg is almost set.

5. Add in the remaining egg, bacon, avocado, and cheese on top of the cooked egg. Let the contents of the pan cook for approximately one minute.

6. Fold the omelet over itself so that the filling is covered. Allow the eggs to cook for another two minutes before removing the omelet from the pan.

7. Serve your omelet with the salsa and enjoy!

2. Baked Eggs and Vegetables

<u>Ingredients</u>

4 Small Asparagus Spears

1 Tbs. of Almond Meal Flour

4 Tbs. of Heavy Whipping Cream

4 tsp. of Parmesan Cheese

2 Large Eggs

A Clove of Garlic, minced

<u>Directions:</u>

1. Heat oven to 400 degrees and prepare a small casserole dish with extra virgin olive oil or baking spray.

2. Next, boil the asparagus for approximately two minutes, until the spears are tender – crisp. Then, drain the vegetables and run them under cold water. Pat the asparagus dry and place in the casserole dish.

3. Pour the heavy cream over top of the asparagus. Now, crack the two eggs on top over the spears.

4. Now, in a bowl, stir the almond flour, cheese, and minced garlic. Sprinkle the mixture over top of the eggs. Put into the oven and bake for six to eight minutes, depending on how you like your eggs.

5. Remove the dish from the oven and enjoy!

3. Ham, Egg, and Garden Vegetable Breakfast Blend

<u>Ingredients</u>

1 ½ Tbs. of Extra Virgin Olive Oil

1 Plum Tomato

2 Tbs. of Butter

½ Medium- Sized Onion, chopped

1 Tbs. of Basil

1 Medium- Sized Bell Pepper

2 Oz. of Ham

3 Large Eggs

1 Clove of Garlic, minced

Directions:

1. Begin by heating the olive oil in skillet on medium heat. Put the onion into the pan and sauté until they are soft. Next, add in the garlic and cook with the onion for approximately one minute.

2. Next, add the peppers and tomatoes into the skillet. Cover the pan and cook the vegetables for ten minutes, until the veggies have softened. Stir the contents of the pan occasionally.

3. Remove lid from pan and have vegetables to simmer until the sauce thickens, stirring frequently.

4. In a bowl, whisk eggs until blended. Then, in a separate skillet, melt butter to layer the bottom. Add in the eggs and basil, and then cook and scramble the eggs until curds form.

5. Add the vegetable mixture and ham into the eggs and stir the contents until the ingredients are mixed together.

6. Remove your breakfast from the pan and enjoy with salt and pepper!

4. Pepper Rings with Egg Filling

Ingredients

2 Tbs. of Shredded Mozzarella Cheese

½ of a Large Red Bell Pepper

2 tbs. of Extra Virgin Olive Oil

2 Large Eggs

Directions:

1. Slice bell pepper across the middle. Next, cut two 1- inch thick rings from the pepper. Carefully use a knife or spoon to remove the ribs and seeds of the pepper rings.

2. Next, put the pepper rings into a skillet with the extra virgin olive oil. Cook over medium heat.

3. Now, crack one egg into each ring and continue to cook until the egg whites are fully set. Do not flip the egg.

4. Sprinkle the shredded mozzarella cheese onto the eggs and cover the skillet. Allow the cheese to melt for one minute, and then season with salt and pepper. Enjoy!

5. Spicy Eggs and Yogurt

<u>Ingredients</u>

2 Large Eggs

1 Tbs. of Chopped Leek

1 tsp. of Lemon Juice

1/3 Cup of Full Fat Greek Yogurt

4 Tbs. of Chopped Scallion

½ Clove of Garlic, halved

½ tsp. of Oregano

¼ Cup of Spinach

2 Tbs. of Butter, divided

1 ½ Tbs. of Extra Virgin Olive Oil

1 Dash of Chili Powder

<u>Directions:</u>

1. Heat your oven to 300 degrees. Begin by combining the yogurt and garlic in a small bowl. Add in a sprinkle of salt, and then set aside.

2. Add one tablespoon of butter and the oil in a skillet and melt on medium heat. Then, add the scallion and leek into the pan and reduce the heat to a lower setting. Continue cooking until the ingredients are soft: approximately ten minutes of cooking time.

3. Next, heat to medium – high and add the spinach and lemon juice into the skillet. Cook the spinach until the leaves have wilted, stirring often.

4. Now, transfer the spinach into a separate skillet, leaving the liquid in the original pan. Then, use a spoon to make deep indentations in the middle of the spinach for the eggs.

5. Crack both eggs into each indentation, and then cook until the egg whites have set: approximately ten minutes.

6. In a pan, liquefy the last tablespoon of butter on medium heat. Add in the remaining unused ingredients and cook until the butter begins to foam.

7. Now, remove the garlic from the yogurt dressing and discard. Dollop the yogurt over the eggs and spinach, and serve with a drizzle of spicy butter. Enjoy!

6. New Way for Bacon and Eggs

Ingredients

1 ½ Oz. of Cream Cheese

1 Pinch of Thyme

2 Large Hard- Boiled Eggs

2 Slices of Bacon

Directions:

1. Heat oven to 400 degrees and coat baking sheet with olive oil spray.

2. Begin preparing the cream cheese filling by combining the thyme and cream cheese in a bowl. Cover filling and put aside for later.

3. Next, peel the hard – boiled eggs, then carefully slice them lengthwise.

4. Use a spoon to remove the yolks from the white halves and discard. Fill two of the egg white halves with the filling, and then use the remaining two to cover the filling.

5. Next, tightly wrap slice of bacon around each of the eggs. Then, place the bacon- wrapped eggs in the baking dish.

6. Bake eggs in oven for thirty minutes. Remove from heat and enjoy!

7. Low- Carb Pancakes

Ingredients

2 Large Eggs

½ tsp. of Cinnamon

2 Oz. of Full Fat Cream Cheese

1 tsp. of Sugar

1 Tbs. of Butter

Directions:

1. Simply combine ingredients with blender; pulse until smooth. Allow the batter to rest for a few minutes as the bubbles settle.
2. Heat the butter in a skillet on medium- high so that it melts as a coating for the bottom of the pan.
3. Next, pour ¼ of the pancake batter into the pan so that it forms the shape of a pancake. Cook until the underside of the pancake is golden brown. Then, flip the cake so that the other side can bake.
4. When the underside has turned golden, remove the pancake from heat and repeat the process until you have used up the rest of the batter. Enjoy!

8. Spinach and Feta Breakfast Quiche

Ingredients

3 Large Eggs

4 Oz. of Button Mushrooms

2 Oz. of Feta Cheese, crumbled

½ Clove of Garlic, minced

5 tsp. of Parmesan Cheese

¼ Cup of Mozzarella Cheese

5 Oz. of Frozen Spinach, thawed

Directions:

1. Heat oven to 350 degrees and prepare a small pie pan with olive oil spray.

2. Start by squeezing the spinach in a paper towel, to remove the excess moisture. Prepare the mushrooms by rinsing them, then thinly slicing them.

3. Place a pan on medium heat, and layer with olive oil spray. Add the mushrooms and garlic into the pan and sauté until mushrooms are soft: approximately 6 minutes.

4. Next, place the spinach into baking dish, followed by the mushrooms. Add the crumbled feta cheese on top of the mushrooms to create a third layer.

5. Beat eggs and parmesan. Then, pour mixture on into the baking dish.

6. Finally, top the quiche with mozzarella cheese, and then put in oven.

7. Bake the quiche for approximately forty minutes, until the top is golden brown. Then, serve and enjoy!

9. Coconut Chia Seed Breakfast Pudding

Ingredients

¼ Cup of Chia Seeds

2 tsp. of Honey

1 Cup of Full Fat Coconut Milk

Directions:

1. Simple combine seeds, honey, and milk in a small bowl. Then, place in the refrigerator overnight.

2. In the morning, remove the bowl from the fridge and enjoy the pudding with a side of your favorite berries.

10. Salmon and Egg Avocados

Ingredients:

2 Large Eggs

1 Avocado

Salt and Pepper

1 Oz. of Smoked Salmon

¼ tsp. of Chili Flakes

Directions:

1. Heat oven to 425 degrees and prepare a sheet with olive oil spray.
2. Slice the avocado in half, lengthwise. Then, remove the seed. Use spoon to remove some of the avocado flesh, so that the holes are big enough for an egg to fit in.
3. Place the avocado halves onto the baking sheet and use the strips of salmon to line the hollows.
4. Crack the eggs into a small bowl, and carefully spoon the yolks and some of the egg whites into the avocado halves.
5. Season your breakfast with spices, and then put in oven. Cook for approximately eighteen minutes.
6. Remove from oven, and then top with the chili flakes. Enjoy!

Chapter 6: 10 Crave- Worthy Lunches

1. Caprese Omega- 3 Salad

Ingredients

¼ Cup of Balsamic Vinegar

½ Cup of Cherry Tomatoes, halved

1 Tbs. of Brown Sugar

2 Oz. of Fresh Mozzarella

4 tsp. of Extra Virgin Olive Oil

1 Avocado, halved, seeded, and diced

2 Cups of Romaine Lettuce, chopped

1 Tbs. of Basil Leaves

1 Boneless, Skinless Chicken Breast, thinly sliced

Directions:

1. Start by preparing the balsamic reduction. Do this by adding the brown sugar and balsamic vinegar into saucepan on medium heat. Allow the sauce to come to a boil, and then lower heat halfway. Cook for approximately seven minutes, and then set aside to cool.

2. Next, in a separate skillet, heat the oil on medium- high heat.

3. Place the chicken breast into the skillet and cook until meat is finished cooking; flipping the chicken once. Allow the chicken to cool before chopping it into cubes.

4. Finally, add the romaine lettuce into a bowl, and add chicken and remaining ingredients. Pour the balsamic vinegar dressing on salad and gently toss. Enjoy!

2. Low- Carb Shrimp Salad

Ingredients

¼ Head of Cauliflower

½ Cucumber

¼ lb. of Raw Shrimp

2 tsp. of Extra Virgin Olive Oil

½ Tbs. of Lemon Zest

1 Tbs. of Chopped Dill

<u>Directions:</u>

1. Preheat your oven to 350 degrees and layer sheet with cooking spray. Begin preparing your salad by peeling and cleaning your shrimp. Additionally, remove the tails as well.

2. Place the shrimp onto the sheet and put into the oven. Cook for eight minutes, until the shrimp is opaque.

3. While the shrimp is cooking, cut the florets off the cauliflower and discard the bottom stalk. Carefully chop the florets into small pieces, then place in a microwave- safe dish.

4. Cook the cauliflower in the microwave for five minutes, so that it is soft, but not mushy.

5. Set aside the shrimp and cauliflower to cool. Then, peel and chop the cucumbers into small pieces.

6. Once cooled, slice the shrimp into halves lengthwise. Then, in a bowl, mix together the all of the ingredients, evenly coating the cauliflower and shrimp with olive oil and lemon juice. Enjoy!

3. Zucchini Protein Pasta

<u>Ingredients</u>

1 Tbs. of Extra Virgin Olive Oil

½ Cup of Cherry Tomatoes

1 Medium Zucchinis

¼ Cup of Sun- Dried Tomatoes

½ Lemon, juiced

½ Cup of Basil, chopped

½ Serving of Vegetable Pasta

1 Oz. of Grated Parmesan Cheese

1 Large Poached Egg

½ Tbs. of Toasted Pine Nuts

Directions:

1. Cook the vegetable pasta in correlation with instructions providing on the packaging. While you are waiting for the pasta to cook, finely dice the cherry tomatoes and transfer them into a bowl.

2. Add the sun- dried tomatoes, garlic, lemon juice, basil, and a sprinkle of red pepper flakes (optional) to the bowl. Then, set the tomato mixture aside and allow to rest for ten minutes.

3. Now, use a spiralizer to spiralize the zucchini to create long noodles that resemble spaghetti. Add the zucchini noodles and veggie noodles into a deep bowl and toss together with oil.

4. Top your pasta with your homemade tomato sauce and poached egg. Sprinkle parmesan cheese on top with the pine nuts, and enjoy!

4. Portabella Mushroom Burgers

Ingredients

2 Portabella Mushroom Caps, stems removed

1 Slice of Halloumi

1 ½ Tbs. of Balsamic Vinegar

1 Thick Slice of Tomato

1 Tbs. of Extra Virgin Olive Oil

Directions:

1. Heat grill to medium heat, and wash and dry your mushroom caps.

2. In a small shallow dish, use a fork to whisk the balsamic vinegar and extra virgin olive oil. Then, place the mushroom caps gill-side down into to the dressing.

3. Next, place the mushrooms on the grill and cook for approximately five minutes; until they start to sweat. Then, flip the mushrooms so that the other side grills for another three minutes.

4. Place the halloumi on the grill and allow to cook for two minutes on both sides, until the cheese is pliable.

5. Start assembling your burger, using the mushroom caps as the bun and the cheese as the patty. Lightly season the tomato and then place the second mushroom on top to create the sandwich. Enjoy!

5. Spaghetti- Inspired Squash Pasta

<u>Ingredients</u>

     1 Spaghetti Squash

     1 Cup of Kale

     ¾ Cup of Chickpeas, cooked

     2 Cloves of Garlic, min

     1 Tbs. of Extra Virgin Olive Oil

     ½ Cup of Toasted Hazelnuts

     2 Tbs. of Parmesan Cheese

<u>Directions:</u>

1. Heat your oven to 400 degrees, and prepare a sheet with olive oil spray.

2. Begin by slicing your spaghetti squash in half lengthwise, then removing the seeds. Rub each half with half a tablespoon of olive oil on the inside of the vegetable.

3. Place the squash facedown onto sheet and put in oven for forty minutes.

4. As the squash is baking, prepare the filling. Start by washing the kale and removing the ribs of the leaves. Then, roughly chop the leaves into small pieces.

5. In a pan, heat oil and minced garlic for two minutes. Add in the kale and continue cooking until the leaves turn bright green and have just started to wilt.

6. Next, add the chickpeas into the skillet and cook until they are warm. Then, transfer pan from heat and put aside.

7. Remove the baking sheet from the oven and use fork to remove the insides of the squash to form strands of spaghetti. Transfer the strands into a bowl, and the mix the spaghetti with the kale mixture.

8. Serve your dish topped with hazelnuts and parmesan cheese. Enjoy!

6. Simple Cucumber Salad

<u>Ingredients</u>

1 Medium Cucumber

1 Pinch of Pink Himalayan Salt

2 Tbs. of Rice Vinegar

1 Tbs. of Toasted Sesame Seeds

½ tsp. of Sugar

<u>Directions:</u>

1. Start by peeling the cucumber, and then slicing it in half lengthwise. Next, use a spoon to scrap out the seeds.

2. Use a knife or carefully slice the cucumber into thin slices. Then, use a double layer of paper towels to gently press the excess moisture from the cucumber slices.

3. In a bowl, mix sugar, vinegar, and salt until the sugar is dissolved.

4. In a medium bowl, toss the cucumbers, sesame seeds, and dressing until the mixture is well combined. Enjoy!

7. Broccoli and Feta Salad

<u>Ingredients</u>

1 Cup of Broccoli Florets, finely chopped

3 Tbs. of Feta Cheese

½ Cup of Chickpeas, rinsed

2 Tbs. of Full Fat Yogurt

3 Tbs. of Chopped Red Bell Pepper

½ Tbs. of Lemon Juice

½ Clove of Garlic, minced

<u>Directions:</u>

1. Start by whisking the feta cheese, garlic, and juice from the lemon in a bowl until the mixture is well combined.

2. Next, add the broccoli, red pepper, and chickpeas into the mixture and toss until evenly coated. Enjoy!

8. Tuna Salad with a Twist

Ingredients

6 Oz. of Chunk Tuna, drained and shredded

¼ Cup of Mayonnaise

½ Cup of Canned Artichoke Hearts

1 tsp. of Lemon Juice

2 Tbs. of Chopped Olives

½ tsp. of Oregano

Directions:

1. For this recipe, all you need to do is mix the ingredients together in a bowl. Enjoy!

9. Squash and Cheese Lunch Cakes

Ingredients

2 Cups of Summer Squash, shredded, seeds removed

1 Large Egg

2/3 Cup of Shallots, chopped

1 Tbs. of Extra Virgin Olive Oil

2 tsp. of Chopped Parsley

4 Tbs. of Parmesan Cheese

Directions:

1. Heat oven to 400 degrees. Begin by whisking the egg in a mixing bowl, then adding the shallots, salt, pepper, and parsley to season.

2. Next, place the shredded squash on a kitchen towel and squeeze out any excess liquid. Then, place the squash and cheese into the bowl that contains the egg mixture and combine.

3. Heat oil in skillet on medium heat and place a quarter of the squash batter onto the pan. Gently pat down the squash so that it forms a small cake. Cook the cake until it is brown and toasted. Then, flip the cake and allow to cook until browned.

4. Remove the squash cake form the skillet and repeat with the rest of the batter.

5. Place all of the cakes onto the skillet and carefully transfer into the oven. Bake for approximately eight minutes, and then serve.

10.   Simple Chickpea Salad

Ingredients

Ranch Dressing:

1 Shallot, peeled

1 Tbs. of Buttermilk Powder

1 Tbs. of White- Wine Vinegar

½ Tbs. of Dill

¼ Cup of Cottage Cheese

2 Tbs. of Mayonnaise

2 Tbs. of Coconut Milk

Salt and Pepper

Chickpea Salad:

1.5 Cups of Cherry Tomatoes, halved

4 Oz. of Chickpeas, rinsed

8 tsp. of Red Onion, chopped

2 Tbs. of Crumbled Feta Cheese

Directions:

1. Start by preparing the dressing. Place the shallot into food processor and process until thinly chopped. Then, add the mayonnaise, buttermilk, cottage cheese, and vinegar into the processor and process smooth.

2. Pour milk in processor as it is running, along with the salt, pepper, and dill.

3. Now, begin preparing the salad but simply combining all of the salad ingredients in a medium bowl. Drizzle dressing in the bowl with the salad ingredients until evenly coated. Enjoy!

Chapter 7: 10 Simple Weight Loss Dinner Ideas

1. Honey Broiled Salmon

Ingredients

    1 Scallion, minced

    ½ lb. Salmon Fillet, skinned

    1 Tbs. of Honey

    2 tsp. of Soy Sauce

    1 Tbs. of Ginger, minced

    1 Tbs. of Rice Vinegar

    1 Clove of Garlic, minced

    ½ tsp. of Toasted Sesame Seeds

Directions:

1. Preheat your broiler and prepare a sheet with olive oil spray.
2. Begin by whisking together the vinegar, ginger, soy sauce, honey, and scallion in a bowl, until the honey has completely dissolved.
3. Next, place the salmon fillet in a sandwich bag and add half of the sauce mixture to marinate the salmon. Seal the plastic bag and place in the refrigerator for fifteen minutes.
4. Once the salmon is finished marinating, place the fillet one to the pan and broil approximately four to six inches away from heat until fully cooked through. This will take about ten minutes.
5. Serve the salmon with a drizzle of the sauce, topped with the sesame seeds. Enjoy!

2. Buffalo Chicken and Artichokes

Ingredients

    1 Large Artichoke, trimmed and prepped

¼ Cup of Shredded Cheddar Cheese

1 Lemon, halved

4 Tbs. of Hot Sauce

¼ lbs. of Cooked Ground Chicken

1 ½ Tbs. of Butter

1 Tbs. of Flour

½ Cup of Coconut Milk

Directions:

1. Begin by bringing pot of water to boil. Then, add the artichoke and lemon to the water, and bring to simmer. Cover pot and let cook for thirty minutes.
2. When the artichoke is finished cooking, transfer from the pot to a kitchen towel to allow the water to drain.
3. Now, preheat your oven to 400 degrees and prepare sheet with spray. Place the artichokes onto the sheet and splay the leaves.
4. Use a spoon to add the ground chicken in between the artichoke layers.
5. Next, liquefy butter in saucepan on medium heat. Add flour and beat with the butter for one minute. In small amount, pour the coconut milk into the saucepan, whisking the mixture until thickened.
6. Remove the saucepan from the stovetop and stir in the hot sauce and cheese.
7. Carefully pour the cheese over top of the artichokes and put in oven for ten minutes. Remove from oven and enjoy!

3. Simple Taco Skillet

Ingredients

½ lb. of Ground Beef

1 Cup of Baby Kale

½ Yellow Onion, diced

Taco Seasoning

1 Bell Pepper, diced

½ Cup of Shredded Cheddar Cheese

½ Can of Diced Tomatoes with Chilies

1 Zucchini, diced

<u>Directions:</u>

1. In a medium pan, brown the beef and crumble. Then, drain the excess grease.
2. Next, add the peppers and onion into the skillet and continue cooking until both vegetables have browned. Then, add in the canned tomatoes, taco seasoning, and as much water as the seasoning packet instructions calls for.
3. Now, add the kale into the taco beef mixture and mix well. Add in the cheese and allow it to melt into the beef, stirring frequently. Once the cheese has melted, remove from heat and enjoy over a bowl of lettuce.

4. Spinach and Artichoke Frittata

<u>Ingredients</u>

3 Large Eggs

1 Shallot, diced

2 Oz. of Marinated Artichokes, diced

1 Tbs. of Extra Virgin Olive Oil

1 Clove of Garlic, minced

4 Broccoli Florets, chopped fine

1 Tbs. of Chives

½ Cup of Spinach

1 Green Onion, finely sliced

2 Tbs. of Feta Cheese

Directions:

1. Coat a skillet with the oil on medium- heat. Add the shallots and garlic into the pan, and sauté for two minutes.
2. Next, add the broccoli into the pan and continue cooking until soft. Then, add in the spinach and stir into the mixture until the leaves have wilted.
3. While the vegetables are cooking, whisk the eggs and chives together in a mixing bowl. Pour the eggs into the vegetables and stir together.
4. Now, add in the artichoke hearts and allow the frittata to cook until the eggs are almost set. Preheat your broiler to 500 degrees.
5. Reduce the heat of the stovetop to medium/ low and continue cooking for an another two minutes. Transfer the skillet to the oven and broil until the frittata is browned.
6. Serve your dinner with crumbled feta cheese and enjoy!

5. Enchilada Zucchini Boats

Ingredients

Sauce:

½ Garlic Clove

¼ Cup of Chicken Broth

½ Tbs. of Hot Sauce

Salt and Pepper

1/3 Cup of Tomato Sauce

A Pinch of Chili Powder and Ground Cumin

Zucchini Boats:

1 Zucchini

¼ Cup of Green Bell Pepper, diced

½ tsp. of Extra Virgin Olive Oil

2 Tbs. of Chopped Cilantro

¼ Cup of Green Onions, diced

1 ½ Tbs. of Water

4 Oz. of Cooked Chicken Breast, shredded

½ Tbs. of Tomato Paste

½ Clove of Garlic, crushed

A Pinch of Cumin, Oregano, and Chili Powder

¼ Cup of Shredded Cheddar Cheese

Directions:

1. For the sauce, coat a saucepan with cooking spray and sauté the garlic. Then, add in the chili powder, broth, tomato sauce, and cumin to the pan and bring to a boil.

2. Reduce heat and let sauce to simmer for about ten minutes. Then, set aside to use later.

3. Now, bring pot of water to boil and preheat your oven to 400 degrees. Prepare a baking dish with cooking spray.

4. Slice the zucchini in half lengthwise and use a spoon to scoop out the inside, so that the shell is ¼ inch thick. Roughly chop the removed flesh and transfer into a small bowl.

5. Place the zucchini halves into the boiling water. Cook the zucchini for one minute, and then carefully remove the halves from the pot.

6. In a skillet, heat oil on medium- low heat. Add the onion, pepper, and garlic into the pan and cook until the onions are translucent.

7. Next, add the zucchini flesh into the skillet with the cilantro, and cook for approximately four minutes. Add the spices, water, and tomato paste into the pan and cook for three more minutes.

8. Now, add the chicken to the skillet and mix with the contents of the pan for a few minutes.

9. Pour half of the enchilada sauce into the baking dish, and then place the zucchini halves onto the dish, with the cut side facing up.

10. Fill the hollowed inside of the zucchinis with the chicken mixture, pressing the meat into the vegetable until filled. Use the rest of the sauce to cover the filled zucchini halves, and then top with cheddar cheese.

11. Cover the baking dish with aluminum foil and place in the oven. Allow to bake for thirty minutes, and serve once the zucchini is cooked through.

6. Pizza Frittata

<u>Ingredients</u>

½ tsp. of Oregano

6 Large Eggs

3 Tbs. of Dry Red Wine

3 Tbs. of Extra Virgin Olive Oil

½ Cup of Half- and Half

½ Cup of Crushed Tomatoes

1 Cup of Hot Pepperoni, chopped

¼ Cup of Parmesan Cheese

3 Oz. of Shredded Mozzarella Cheese

1 Clove of Garlic, chopped

1 tsp. of Hot Sauce

1 Tbs. of Grated Onion

1 tsp. of Chopped Parsley

<u>Directions:</u>

1. Heat oven to 400 degrees. Begin by whisking the eggs, cream, hot sauce, and parmesan cheese in a bowl.
2. Next, heat ½ of the oil in a pan on medium- high heat. Add the eggs into the pan and move them frequently until they start to firm.
3. Place the skillet into the oven and bake for approximately seven minutes.
4. In a separate skillet, heat remaining oil on medium- high heat and add cook the garlic, onion, and oregano for three minutes. Pour the wine into the pan and slightly reduce the heat.

5. Add the tomatoes into the skillet and simmer for ten minutes, until the sauce has thickened.

6. Remove the skillet from the oven and pour the tomato sauce over top. Sprinkle with mozzarella cheese and place into the oven once again for ten minutes. Top your frittata with parsley and enjoy!

7. Classic Chicken Wings

Ingredients

 1 lb. of Wings and Drumettes

 ½ Tbs. of Butter

 1 Tbs. of Thyme

 3 Garlic Cloves, crushed

 ¼ Cup of Hot Sauce

 For Dip:

  ½ Cup of Greek Yogurt

  ¼ Cup of Blue Cheese Crumbles

Directions:

1. Heat oven to 375 degrees and prepare a baking sheet with cooking spray.
2. In a medium bowl, season the chicken with salt and pepper.
3. Over low heat, melt butter in pan. Add in the garlic and thyme, and let simmer for two minutes. Then, add in the hot sauce, stirring the ingredients together.
4. Pour the hot sauce mixture over the chicken and toss well to evenly coat. Let the wings marinate in the refrigerator for a half hour.
5. While the wings are marinating, begin making your dressing. Simply combine the blue cheese and yogurt together in a bowl, and refrigerate for later.
6. Place the wings and drummettes onto the baking sheet and transfer to the oven. Bake for thirty minutes. Turn the chicken over, and baste with more hot sauce. Then, bake for an additional twenty- five minutes.

7. Remove wings from oven and let to cool before serving with the blue cheese dip. Enjoy!

8. Easy Steak Rolls

<u>Ingredients</u>

½ lb. of Flank Steak

½ Cup of Green Beans

¼ Cup of Steak Marinade

¼ White Onion, sliced into strips

½ Red Bell Pepper, sliced into strips

1 Tbs. of Extra Virgin Olive Oil

<u>Directions:</u>

1. First, marinade your steak in a plastic sandwich bag for thirty minutes with the steak marinade. While your steak is marinating, preheat your oven to 350 degrees and prepare a baking sheet with cooking spray.
2. Next, heat a skillet over medium heat and heat the olive oil in the pan.
3. Slice the steaks in halves. Take a little bit of the peppers, green beans, and onion slices, and tightly wrap the steak slices around the vegetables. Use toothpicks to secure the wrap.
4. Now, add the steak rolls to the skillet and sear for one minute on all sides of the wrap.
5. Carefully transfer the steak rolls onto the baking sheet and place in the oven. Cook for ten minutes, and then remove from the oven. Enjoy!

9. Simple Stuffed Chicken

<u>Ingredients</u>

1 Boneless, Skinless Chicken Breast

2 Oz. of Fresh Mozzarella, sliced

3 Oz. of Roasted Red Peppers, sliced into small pieces

2 Basil Leaves

2 Tbs. of Parmesan Cheese

½ Tbs. of Italian Dressing

Directions:

1. Heat oven to 400 degrees, and prepare a baking dish with cooking spray.
2. Use a knife to butterfly the chicken, cutting the breast lengthwise with about ¼ of an inch from the other side.
3. Spread the chicken breast into the dish, so that you can stuff it. Use salt and pepper to season the chicken.
4. Simply layer the roasted red pepper, and mozzarella cheese onto one side of the chicken. Carefully fold the other half over top, tucking in the stuffed ingredients snuggly into the chicken.
5. Drizzling the Italian dressing over top of the chicken, then place the dish into the oven. Bake for thirty to thirty- five minutes, until the chicken is full cooked.
6. Remove chicken from oven, and turn on your broiler to a high setting. Add any remaining mozzarella cheese and parmesan cheese onto the chicken and place into the oven once more.
7. Broil until the cheese turned golden brown, then remove from heat. Enjoy!

10. **Cauliflower Rice**

Ingredients

1 Cup of Cauliflower

2 tsp. of Soy Sauce

¼ Cup of Onion, chopped

¼ Cup of Baby Carrots, chopped

1 Tbs. of Extra Virgin Olive Oil

¼ Cup of Thawed Frozen Peas

1 Egg, beaten lightly

1 Green Onion, chopped

½ tsp. of Sesame Oil

½ Cup of Bean Sprouts

Directions:

1. Slice the bottom of the cauliflower off, and then cut the cauliflower into florets. Dry off excess water.
2. Place the florets into a food processor and pulse until you achieve the consistency of rice.
3. Next, heat half of oil in skillet on medium- high heat. Add in the onion and fry until it is light brown. Transfer the onions into a bowl and set aside for later.
4. In a small mixing bowl, whisk the egg with the sesame oil and soy sauce. Add a bit more olive oil into the skillet, then quickly scramble the eggs.
5. Transfer the scrambled eggs from the skillet to the bowl with the onion.
6. Add the rest of the olive oil into the skillet and place the cauliflower, green onions, carrots, bean sprouts, and peas in the pan. Stir fry the ingredients for three minutes, then reduce to a lower heat setting.
7. Add in more soy sauce if desired, then cover until the cauliflower is good all the way through. Add the egg and cooked onions into the skillet once more and allow the ingredients to cook together for two minutes.
8. Serve and enjoy!

Conclusion

I hope this book was able to help you to understand the Atkins diet, as well as feel inspired to begin the first phase right now!

The next step is to make the decision to create a better life for yourself by changing your eating habits. You can have the body of your dreams and the greatest health you are able to achieve just by following this intensive meal plan. Health is the most valuable gift you could ever give yourself.

Finally, if you enjoyed this book, please take the time to share your thoughts and post a review on Amazon. It'd be greatly appreciated!

Thank you and good luck!

www.ingramcontent.com/pod-product-compliance
Lightning Source LLC
Chambersburg PA
CBHW072136280526
45788CB00002B/664